D0098200

CANCER
&
Nutrition

CANCER & Nutrition

CHARLES B. SIMONE, M.M.S., M.D.

McGraw-Hill Book Company

New York St. Louis San Francisco Auckland Bogotá Guatemala Hamburg Johannesburg Lisbon London Madrid Mexico Montreal New Delhi Panama Paris San Juan São Paulo Singapore Sydney Tokyo Toronto

1 2 3 4 5 6 7 8 9 0 FGR FGR 8 7 6 5 4 3

ISBN 0-07-057466-9

LIBRARY OF CONGRESS CATALOGING IN PUBLICATION DATA

Simone, Charles B.
Cancer and nutrition.
1. Cancer—Nutritional aspects. 2. Cancer—Prevention. I. Title.
RC262.S53 1983 616.99'4052 82–22948
ISBN 0–07–057466–9

Book design by Nancy Dale Muldoon

Contents

FOUR: MODIFYING THE RISKS

To my family

Foreword

WHEN asked what they fear the most, 65 percent of Americans say cancer. This dread disease is the number two killer in the United States. Because of the nature of the disease, and also because of the drastic methods currently needed for effective treatment—surgery, radiotherapy, and chemotherapy—incredible suffering is experienced by Americans and peoples throughout the world as a consequence of cancer. With control of infections as a cause of disease, suffering, and death, cancer and the other diseases associated with aging—including heart and blood vessel disease—become more and more prominent in our lives. Now even in China, a developing country, cancer and heart disease vie for the number one position as killer of human beings. We all pray for the day when we will understand cancer and doctors can give us a cure, such as the antibiotics we have to treat tuberculosis, pneumonia, and meningitis. That day will come, and hopefully very soon. But since many discoveries will be needed, we can't count on it in our immediate future.

Too few of us realize that the tremendous increase in cancer as a killer of Americans can be halted. Perhaps the measures are too simple. In this refreshingly straightforward book, which is so easy to read, Dr. Simone summarizes current knowledge that promises prevention of many, if not most, cancers. We must stop smoking of all kinds, but especially we must quit smoking cigarettes; indeed, we must avoid completely the use of tobacco. We must exercise regularly, eat a prudent diet, avoid known cancer-causing chemicals, and take rational amounts of certain vitamins and minerals. We must insist that our work places are safe from exposure to known and possibly hazardous chemicals. It even seems most healthful to develop lasting love relationships. These are simple means—all—but abundant experimental epidemiological and clinical evidence indicates that these relatively minor adjustments of life-style, initiated as early in life as possible, could reduce the frequency of cancer dramatically.

Why don't we all make these relatively minor changes in our life-style? I have asked myself this question over and over again. I guess it is because as a species, knowing full well that we are mortal, we have the need to deny our mortality and pretend we are immortal for as long as possible. I took Simone's little test for cancer risks and came out with flying colors—only a very few adjustments still to make. Unfortunately, perhaps I have made many of the changes in life-style a bit late, but I am convinced that if everyone could read Simone's book early enough in life and take it seriously, we would make major strides toward putting the cancer doctors out of work and approach the legacy of health that is within our reach.

ROBERT A. GOOD, PH.D., M.D.
Former President and Director,
Memorial Sloan-Kettering Cancer Hospital,
New York City;
head of Cancer Research Program,
Oklahoma Medical Research Foundation,
Oklahoma City, Oklahoma

Introduction

CANCER is the most feared of all diseases. People immediately associate cancer with dying. Unlike other killer diseases, cancer usually causes a slow death involving pain, suffering, mental anguish, and a feeling of hopelessness. It is the second most common cause of death in the United States and will affect one out of every three or four Americans during their lifetime. The number of new cases of some cancers has been increasing over the past eight decades; the accelerated rise in lung cancer, for example, is alarming. According to the U.S. Bureau of the Census, in 1900, 64 people out of 100,000 died of cancer, making it the sixth leading cause of death. Today, 187 people out of every 100,000 will die of cancer, ranking it second.

Over the past half century, there has been limited progress in the treatment of cancer. In 1971 the United States declared war on cancer with the following statement from President Nixon: "The time has come in America when the same kind of concentrated effort that split the atom and took man to the moon should be turned toward conquering this dread disease." In that year 337,000 people died of cancer, and about $250 million were spent on cancer research. In 1981, ten years and several billion research dollars later, about 420,000 cancer victims died, a 25 percent increase.

Cancer research and treatment are extremely complex fields of study because the exact nature of the single cancer cell is so elusive. Cancer is many diseases with many different causes. One cannot expect miracle cures just because so much money has been poured into research. At the same time, one should not expect miracles from "cancer-cure" facilities that take money from cancer victims desperate to try any treatment in hope of another chance at life.

There is good evidence that 70 to 80 percent of all cancers are produced by diet and nutrition, life-style (smoking, alcohol, etc.), chemicals, and other events in the environment. Since most cancers are induced by nutrition, life-style, and environmental factors, many of these cancers can be eliminated or substantially reduced in number if the risk factors are identified and then modified by an individual to lessen his risk. Many people have the fatalistic attitude that "anything and everything can cause cancer so what's the use in trying to do anything about it?" That attitude is unwarranted and fosters even more apathy. Everything does *not* cause cancer.

The Dietary Goals for the United States, published by the Senate Select Committee on Nutrition and Human Needs (Senator George McGovern, chairman), states that Americans eat too much and, specifically, they eat too much meat, too much fat, too much cholesterol, too much sugar, and too much salt. They should eat more fruits, vegetables, and grains. The committee recommended that current fat consumption, which comprises 40 to 45 percent of the calories in the present American diet, should be reduced to about 30 percent; that sugar calories be reduced to 15 percent from the current 15 to 25 percent, and that salt consumption should be substantially reduced.

The type of diet we eat today and its preparation are proving to be a major risk factor in the development of certain cancers, a risk factor that can definitely be modified. Nutrition is a very complex topic, not well understood by the public or even by some physicians. Americans need to know how nutrition is related to major diseases, based on the presently available information. Diet and nutrition appear to be related to the largest number of human cancers; tobacco smoking is related to about 30 to 40 percent of human cancers. Other known risk factors associated with the development of cancer are alcohol, age, immune system deficiencies, chemicals, and drugs. Having one or more of these risk factors does not mean that cancer necessarily will develop. It simply means that a person with risk factors has a greater than normal chance of developing cancer.

It is the individual's responsibility to learn about the risk factors involved in cancer development and then modify those risk factors accordingly. If cancer prevention is to be achieved, each individual should have his or her own anticancer plan based on risk-factor modification. In addition, your family, and particularly your children, should be taught about risk-factor modification. If nutritional and other risk factors are modified, the benefit will be evident in all people, but especially in the young and in following generations. Obviously some risk factors cannot be controlled by an individual, and there the community must also have its own anticancer plan for the environment.

The Biometry Branch of the National Cancer Institute estimates that between $30 and $35 billion were spent in 1980 for direct and indirect aspects of cancer care (hospitalizations, office visits, loss of time from jobs, research, training, etc.). Over $52 billion were spent in 1980 for cardiovascular disease patients. (Cardiovascular diseases have many risk factors in common with cancer.) In addition, consumers spend billions of dollars each year on quack remedies, get-healthy-quick schemes, and on practitioners and "health" centers which claim to reverse or eliminate chronic diseases easily and quickly. These costs are exorbitant, unreasonable, and place a heavy burden on our economy. We must eliminate or modify all known risk factors so that we will eventually be able to more effectively prevent cancer and heart disease. Nutritional factors and tobacco smoking, for example, are major risk factors to health which if modified or eliminated could dramatically reduce the number of cancer victims as well as heart disease victims. Our health-care system emphasizes expensive medical technology and hospital care. It does not emphasize preventive medicine and health education. *It is your responsibility to learn and modify these risk factors.* Good health does not come easily; you must work for it. Common sense is the major requirement.

ONE

Cancer Today

1

The Scope of Cancer

ONE of every three or four Americans will develop cancer during his or her lifetime.[1] Second only to cardiovascular disease as the leading cause of death in the United States, cancer accounted for 20 percent of all deaths in 1983, with 440,000 mortalities.[2] If present trends continue, the American Cancer Society projects that 510,000 people in the United States will die of cancer by the year 2000.[3] This figure does not even include an estimated 400,000 patients with nonmelanoma skin cancers.[4] Other than the skin, the three organs of the body most affected by cancer are the lungs, the colon and rectum, and the breasts. Table I shows the estimated incidence of cancer in various sites in the body (male and female) and the estimated percent of deaths in each category.

Carcinoma *in situ* of the cervix and skin cancers other than melanoma (a deadly skin cancer) have not been included in the statistics. If they were, the percentages in Table I would be much higher for skin and uterine cancers. The word "incidence" means the *number of newly diagnosed cases of a specific disease,* not the number of deaths. For example, in the United States, the estimated incidence, or number of new cases, of breast cancer in 1983 is 114,900: 900 male and 114,000 female cases. The estimated mortality, or number of deaths, from

Table I*

1983 ESTIMATED CANCER INCIDENCE AND DEATH FOR EACH SITE AND SEX

Organ Site	% Incidence Male	% Incidence Female	% Deaths Male	% Deaths Female
Skin	2	2	2	1
Mouth structure	4	2	3	1
Lung	22	9	35	17
Breast		26		18
Colon & rectum	14	15	12	15
Pancreas	3	3	5	5
Prostate	18		10	
Ovary & uterus		17		11
Urinary tract	9	4	5	3
Blood & lymph glands	8	7	8	9
All other	20	15	20	20

* From Silverberg (1983). See References.

breast cancer in 1983 is 37,500: 300 male and 37,200 female deaths.

The death rate for lung cancer has been rising for both the male and the female population since 1940, and the rate of rise for females is much greater now than ever before. By contrast, since 1930 the death rate has been decreasing for cancer of the uterus, stomach cancer for male and female, and female colon and rectum cancer. However, for some cancers, the death rate has remained approximately the same since 1930,[5] which indicates that little or no real progress has been made in increasing survival in these cancers (breast cancer, ovarian cancer, leukemia, male bladder cancer, prostate cancer, male colon and rectum cancer, and male esophageal cancer). This information is quite disturbing because it indicates that there is no effective treatment for the three cancers that cause 50 percent of all cancer deaths (lung cancer, which has an increasing death rate, colon and rectum cancer, and breast cancer).

These statistics concern the United States as a whole. When each state is examined individually, we find that the states in the northeast and other heavily industrialized states have the highest number of deaths due to cancer. Figure 1 illustrates the cancer death rates geographically, from those states with the most deaths due to cancer to those with the least. Table II lists the states in decreasing order of mortality due to cancer, the actual cancer death rate per 100,000 population, and the total number of deaths in the year compared with the total number of newly diagnosed cancer cases in the year. These

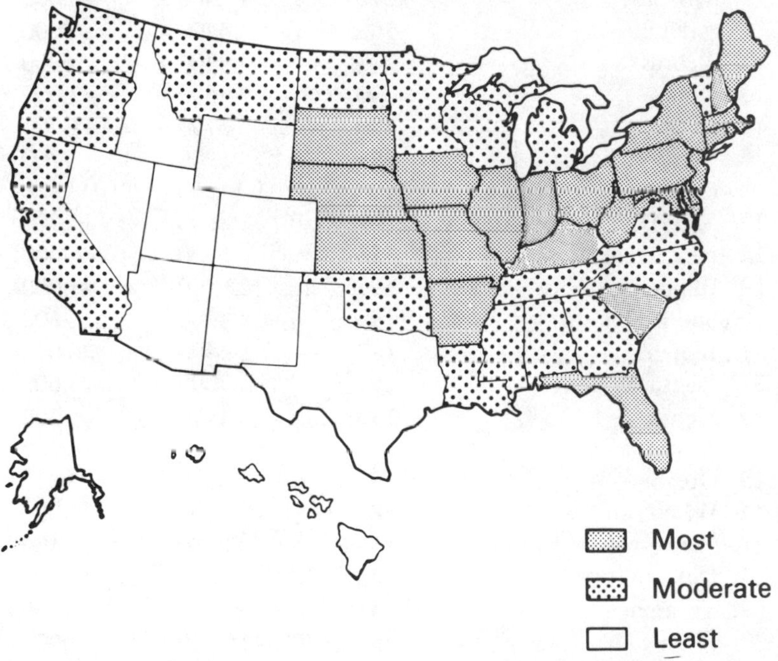

Figure 1. Cancer death rate in the United States—1983

Table II

1983 ESTIMATED CANCER DEATHS BY INCIDENCE RATES IN STATES

State	Death Rate per 100,000	Number of Deaths	Number of New Cases
1. District of Columbia	260	1600	3200
2. Rhode Island	248	2400	4700
3. Florida	237	26,600	51,000
4. Pennsylvania	227	27,000	53,000
5. New Jersey	219	16,400	32,000
6. Maine	217	2500	4800
7. Massachusetts	215	12,600	24,000
8. New York	212	37,500	74,000
9. Connecticut	210	6700	13,000
10. Missouri	210	10,500	20,000
11. Arkansas	203	4700	9000
12. Nebraska	201	3200	6000
13. Ohio	200	21,500	42,000
14. Iowa	199	5700	11,200
15. West Virginia	199	3900	7700
16. Delaware	198	1200	2400
17. Maryland	197	8600	16,700
18. New Hampshire	196	1900	3600
19. Illinois	195	22,500	44,000
20. South Dakota	193	1300	2600
21. Indiana	192	10,400	20,000
22. Kentucky	191	7000	13,600
23. Kansas	190	4600	8700
24. Alabama	186	7400	14,300
25. Oregon	186	5000	9800
26. Wisconsin	186	9000	18,000
27. Tennessee	184	8600	17,100
28. Oklahoma	183	6000	11,600
29. Vermont	181	950	2000
30. Michigan	181	16,400	32,000
31. Mississippi	180	4600	8900
32. North Dakota	179	1200	2500

1983 ESTIMATED CANCER DEATHS BY INCIDENCE RATES IN STATES—*Continued*

State	Death Rate per 100,000	Number of Deaths	Number of New Cases
33. Minnesota	177	7300	14,000
34. California	175	44,500	85,000
35. North Carolina	170	10,400	20,000
36. Louisiana	167	7600	14,800
37. Washington	165	7300	14,400
38. Arizona	165	4900	9000
39. Montana	162	1300	2600
40. Virginia	158	8900	17,200
41. Georgia	155	9000	17,300
42. South Carolina	150	4900	9600
43. Idaho	141	1400	2700
44. Texas	140	22,400	44,000
45. Nevada	136	1300	2600
46. New Mexico	129	1800	3500
47. Colorado	124	3900	7600
48. Wyoming	120	650	1300
49. Hawaii	118	1200	2400
50. Utah	91	1500	3000
51. Alaska	69	300	600

data are not age adjusted, which means that the figures do not reflect whether the population in the state is evenly distributed according to age. For example, Florida, a state not in the industrial northeast, has the third highest cancer death rate in the country (237 cancer deaths for every 100,000 population in the state). The reason is that so many of our senior citizens retire to Florida.

Table III shows nations of the world and their order in rank according to cancer death rates from highest to lowest. Uruguay has the highest cancer death rate for both men and

Table III

CANCER IN THE WORLD*

	Male Deaths	Female Deaths
1.	Uruguay	Uruguay
2.	Scotland	Denmark
3.	Belgium	Scotland
4.	Netherlands	Hungary
5.	Hungary	Ireland
6.	France	England & Wales
7.	England & Wales	Austria
8.	Austria	W. Germany
9.	W. Germany	Chile
10.	Singapore	New Zealand
11.	Switzerland	Northern Ireland
12.	Denmark	Belgium
13.	Northern Ireland	Netherlands
14.	Hong Kong	Israel
15.	Ireland	Sweden
16.	New Zealand	Costa Rica
17.	United States	Iceland
18.	Poland	Argentina
19.	Argentina	United States
20.	East Germany	Canada

* Nations ranked in order of age-adjusted cancer death rates per 100,000 population based on information from 1976–1977.

There were no statistics available for the Soviet Union or most of its satellite nations.

Statistics from the People's Republic of China show that it has much less cancer than the above countries.[6]

women. The United States is ranked seventeenth highest in the world for male cancer deaths and nineteenth highest for female cancer deaths. There were no statistics available for the Soviet Union or most of its satellite nations.

2

Risk Factors—An Overview

DIET AND NUTRITIONAL RISK FACTORS

DIET and/or nutritional deficiencies are now strongly correlated with many cancers (see Table I). The National Academy of Sciences and Wynder and Gori estimate that nutritional factors account for 60 percent of women's and 40 percent of men's cancers.[1,2,3] Cancers of the breast, uterus, kidney, and colon are closely associated with consumption of total protein and total fat, particularly meat and animal fat. Other cancers that are directly correlated with dietary factors are cancers of the rectum, stomach, small intestine, mouth, pharynx, esophagus, pancreas, liver, ovary, endometrium, prostate, thyroid, and bladder.[4,5,6,7,8,9] Aflatoxin, a fungus product which is found on certain edible plants (especially peanuts) is related to human liver cancer.[10,11] Recently, excessive consumption of coffee has been correlated with cancer of the pancreas,[12] but considerable doubt has been cast upon this correlation.[13,14] These cancers and their relation to diet and nutritional factors will be discussed in separate chapters.

CHEMICAL AND ENVIRONMENTAL RISK FACTORS

Chemical and environmental factors, including diet and lifestyle, may be responsible for causing 70 to 80 percent of all

Table I

CANCER RISK FACTORS

Risk Factor	Site of Human Cancer
1. *Diet or nutritional deficiencies*	
In general	Breast, colon, rectum, stomach, mouth, pharynx, esophagus, pancreas, liver, ovary, endometrium, prostate, thyroid, kidney, bladder
Iodine deficiency	Thyroid, breast
Aflatoxin (fungus product)	Liver
Coffee—excessive consumption	Pancreas?
2. *Tobacco smoking, chewing, etc.*	Lung, larynx, mouth, pharynx, esophagus, pancreas, bladder, kidney
3. *Alcohol*	Mouth, pharynx, esophagus, gastrointestine, pancreas, liver, head and neck, larynx, bladder
4. *Age* greater than 55	Many organ sites
5. *Immune system malfunction*	Lymphoma, carcinoma
6. *High blood pressure*	Breast, colon
7. *Obesity*	Breast, endometrium
8. *Hormonal*	
Late/never pregnant	Breast
Fibrocystic breast disease	Breast
DES (diethylstilbestrol)	Breast, vagina, cervix, endometrium, testicle
Conjugated estrogens	Breast, liver
Androgens (17-methyl subst)	Liver

CANCER RISK FACTORS—*Continued*

Risk Factor	Site of Human Cancer
Undescended testicles (especially after age 6)	Testicle
9. *Sexual-Social*	
Female promiscuity	Uterine cervix
Poor male hygiene	Penis
Male homosexuality (promiscuity, amyl nitrite)	Kaposi's sarcoma, anus, tongue
10. *Radiation*	
X-rays, etc. (ionizing)	Skin, breast, myelogenous leukemia, thyroid, bone
Sunlight (UV) excessive in fair-skinned people who burn easily	Skin
11. *Occupational*	
Petroleum, tar, soots	Lung, skin, scrotum
Boot and shoe manufacture and repair	Nasal sinus
Furniture and cabinetmaking industry	Nasal sinus
Rubber industry	Lung, bladder, leukemia, stomach
Chemists	Brain, lymphoma, leukemia, pancreas
Foundry workers	Lung
Painters	Leukemia
Printing workers	Lung, mouth, pharynx
Textile workers	Nasal sinus

cancers. Theoretically, then, most cancers could be prevented if the factors which cause them can first be identified and then controlled or eliminated. Throughout their lives, people are exposed to many chemicals and some drugs in small amounts and in many combinations unique to their culture and environment. Many chemicals and drugs are now known to cause human cancer and many more are suspected.[15] Table II lists chemicals, their uses, and the human cancers associated with them. People who are exposed to these chemicals either directly (those who work in the particular industry shown) or indirectly (for example, firefighters exposed to burning objects made from these chemicals) are at increased risk of developing the cancer listed in the table. The incidence of certain cancers in particular populations reflects prolonged low-level exposure to many carcinogens (chemical substances which cause cancer), cocarcinogens (substances which activate carcinogens), and promoting factors (substances which facilitate the action of carcinogens).

The mortality rate from lung cancer has been increasing for the past fifteen years, even though it has been known throughout that period that cigarette smoking is the major cause of the disease. It has been estimated that 40 percent of all cancers may be related to smoking, either directly or indirectly. The incidence of cancers of the lung, head and neck, esophagus, pancreas, kidney, and bladder is increased in people who smoke. The fifteen carcinogens which have been found in tobacco smoke include hydrocarbons and aromatic amines. People who work with asbestos or uranium or who drink alcohol have an increased risk and incidence of getting cancer if they also smoke. (This is called synergism, an action of two or more substances achieving a result of which each substance individually is incapable.) It seems reasonable then to explore ways to decrease the number of cancers related to smoking and other known human carcinogens by reducing the number of new smokers, encouraging current smokers to quit, and

Table II

DRUG AND CHEMICAL CANCER RISK FACTORS

Risk Factor	Use	Site of Cancer
1. *Drugs*		
Chlorambucil	Anticancer	Leukemia
Chloramphenicol	Antibiotic	Leukemia
Cyclophosphamide	Anticancer	Bladder
Dilantin	Anticonvulsant	Lymph tissue
Melphalan	Anticancer	Leukemia
Phenacetin	Relieves pain	Kidney
Thiotepa	Anticancer	Leukemia
2. *Chemicals*		
Acrylonitrile	Raw material for synthetic fibers, rubbers, resins, and pharmaceutical, dyes, and surfactants	Lung
4-Aminobiphenyl	Organic rubber, dyes	Bladder
Aniline	Manufacture of dyes, pharmaceutical, photographic chemicals, rubber, herbicides, fungicides	Bladder
Arsenic	Alloy additive, certain glass, doping agent in silicon solid state, some solders, in some drinking water	Skin, lung, liver
Asbestos	Insulation, cements, brake lining, fireproofing gloves and clothes	Lung, pleura, gastrointestine
Auramine (mfgr)	Dye for paper, textile, leather, corrugated cardboard; antiseptic	Bladder

DRUG AND CHEMICAL CANCER RISK FACTORS—*Cont.*

Risk Factor	Use	Site of Cancer
Benzene	Manufacture of medicine, chemicals, dyes, insecticides, paint remover, rubber cement, antiknock gasoline	Acute myelogenous leukemia
Benzidene	Dyes, some rubbers, detects blood	Bladder
Beryllium	TV phosphors, computer parts, aerospace industry, rocket fuels, alloy	Lung
Cadmium industry	Electroplating, alloys, electrical equipment, solar batteries, fire protection, TV phosphors, pigments, rubber and plastics, control of atomic fission in reactors, fungicide	Prostate, lung
Carbon tetrachloride	Solvent, refrigerant and propellant, semiconductors, fumigant	Liver
Chlormethyl Ether	Solvent, refrigerant	Lung
Chloroprene	Manufacture of synthetic rubber	Skin, lung, liver
Chromate	Catalyst, chromium plating, tanning, pigments, pharmaceuticals	Lung, nasal sinus
Isopropyl alcohol (acid process)	Intermediate for solvent, antifreeze, preservative; perfume; cosmetic	Nasal sinus, larynx

DRUG AND CHEMICAL CANCER RISK FACTORS—*Cont.*

Risk Factor	Use	Site of Cancer
Mustard gas	Pharmaceutical industry	Lung, larynx
Nickel	Raw material for alloy, alkali batteries, ceramics, coins	Nasal sinus, lung
Hematite mining (radon?)	Paints, abrasives, metals, pharmaceuticals	Lung
Vinyl chloride	Plastics, cooling medium	Lung, liver, brain

by eliminating the other carcinogens altogether from our diet or eliminating our exposure to them.

It is known that not all people exposed to a carcinogen have the same probability of getting cancer. This is because certain proteins from the liver, called enzymes, can break down or activate the carcinogen at different speeds in different people to either render it harmless or promote it to cause cancer. This is related to genetics; these enzymes will either destroy or activate carcinogens to varying degrees according to inherited tendencies. Some foods can induce certain enzymes to destroy certain carcinogens. The most potent food sources to induce these enzymes are vegetables of the *Brassicaceae* family, which includes Brussels sprouts, cabbage, and broccoli.[16]

Environmental factors, on the other hand, may be just as important as genetic factors. For example, whereas Japanese men and women who leave Japan and settle in Hawaii or the continental United States have a decreased risk of getting stomach cancer, those who remain in Japan have a high incidence of stomach cancer. Stomach cancer in the United States has steadily been decreasing with the advent of refrigeration, because refrigeration decreases the carcinogen called nitrosamine, which is formed from nitrite food preservatives.

OCCUPATIONAL RISK FACTORS

About 10 percent of all cancers are related to occupational exposure. The relationship between a man's occupation and cancer was noted in the eighteenth century when it was observed that the incidence of cancer of the scrotum was very high in chimney sweeps. Many associations between exposure to carcinogens at work and cancer have been made since then. Most recently, the boot and shoe manufacture and repair industry and the furniture and cabinetmaking industry were shown to be risk factors for developing cancer of the nasal sinuses.[17]

Preliminary studies indicate that butchers and slaughterhouse workers are at risk for developing lung cancer and cancer of other parts of the respiratory system as well as some leukemias.[18,19] However, these findings need to be confirmed and controlled for those persons who also smoke before this industry can be labeled as a definite risk factor for cancer.

AGE AS A RISK FACTOR

The older a person gets the higher is his or her risk of developing cancer. The risk is not as high as the increased risk for cardiovascular disease, however. The Biometry Section of the National Cancer Institute has presented studies which show that with every five-year increase of age there is a doubling in the incidence of cancer.[20] The elderly often suffer from nutritional deficiencies, and they have an increased number of infections, autoimmune diseases, and infantile disease patterns, as well as cancer. Werner's syndrome, which prematurely ages very young children so that they all die in early adolescence, is characterized by an impaired immune system. These facts suggest that the immune system (see Chapter 4) in the elderly is not working properly.[21] This is related in part to poor nutrition. In addition, it seems that age provides the necessary amount of time for many external events to occur to the body which lead eventually to the development of cancer. That is, it is not the age of a person alone that causes cancer, but rather it is the time the person has been exposed to so many external risk factors and events. A good example of this is lung cancer in cigarette smokers. The longer the person is exposed to smoking, the greater the likelihood and incidence of lung cancer. For men between 55 and 64, the annual lung cancer mortality rate is five times higher if they started to smoke before age 15 than if they started to smoke after age 25.[22] If a person stops smoking, there is a decreased risk in developing lung cancer, but this risk does not go back to zero.

GENETIC RISK FACTORS

Cancer is usually characterized by abnormal genetic chromosome material in the affected cancer cell. A cancer cell does not have the proper amount or type of genes, or more specifically, DNA (deoxyribonucleic acid) content. People with certain inherited diseases are more prone to getting cancer. There are over 200 genetic conditions which have an increased incidence of cancer,[23] including mongolism or trisomy 21 syndrome, the immunodeficiency syndromes, Gardner's syndrome, and many more. These genetic abnormalities, although important for the physician to recognize, account for only a small fraction of all human cancer.

ATHEROSCLEROSIS AND CANCER

Atherosclerosis and its many complications are the most common cause of death in the United States. Atherosclerosis, commonly called "hardening of the arteries," is a disease which narrows the inside diameter of the artery. This narrowing restricts the blood flow beyond the narrowed portion and therefore delivers less oxygen to those tissues since oxygen is carried by red blood cells. Death of tissues results directly from low or no oxygen. The less oxygen, the more dead tissue. Pain is a symptom of either very low oxygen delivered to tissues or outright death of tissues. This is why when a person is having a "heart attack," he has a lot of pain: some tissues are dying and others are not receiving enough oxygen. What does atherosclerosis have to do with cancer? Well, cancer may be responsible for the development of heart and vessel disease in a way, and high blood pressure (a form of blood vessel disease) may lead to the development of cancer under certain circumstances.

The first step in the formation of a narrowed artery is the manufacture of cells (smooth muscle cells) which line the inside of the artery. Then cholesterol gets deposited in these cells after they have increased in number. The increased cells together with cholesterol is called a plaque. There is good evidence that these cells come from a single cell, that is, they are cloned from one common cell. Cloning is a form of cancer.[24] This situation can be produced in chickens by feeding them carcinogens benzo(a)pyrene and dimethylbenzanthracene), chemical substances that produce cancer. These particular carcinogens cause an increase in the number and rate of formation of plaques without altering the blood level of cholesterol. In humans, these types of carcinogens (hydrocarbons) are carried by certain proteins (low-density lipoproteins) which also carry cholesterol. More curiously, an enzyme called aryl hydrocarbon hydroxylase, present in cells of the inner walls of arteries, can activate hydrocarbon carcinogens to start proliferating the lining cells.[25] Therefore, if we eat food contaminated with these hydrocarbons or are otherwise exposed to them so that they get into our bloodstream, atherosclerosis may begin to develop. Of course this is just one of many factors involved in the development of atherosclerosis.

R. W. Pero and colleagues have shown a relationship between high blood pressure and cancer.[26] The study shows that the higher the blood pressure and the older the person, the more DNA alterations occur in cells. The more abnormal the DNA content of a cell, the more often it will lose control and develop into a cancer. There is some evidence that people with high blood pressure are at an increased risk of developing breast cancer,[27] colon cancer, lung cancer, and other cancers.[28]

HORMONAL RISK FACTORS

Hormones influence a cell's growth and development, and if hormones are in excess or deficit inside the body, then cells will not function properly and may grow abnormally or aberrantly and become cancer cells.

Women who have never been pregnant have a higher risk of developing breast cancer than women who do have children; and women who become pregnant before age 20 have a reduced risk. Women whose mothers or other close relatives have breast cancer have three times the normal risk of getting breast cancer. Women who do not menstruate during their lifetime have a three to four times higher risk of developing breast cancer after the age of 55. A lower risk of breast cancer is seen in women whose ovaries cease to function or are removed surgically before age 35.

There has been considerable controversy as to whether birth control pills can cause breast and liver cancer. It appears from several studies that hormones used in birth control pills are a risk factor for causing breast or liver cancer;[29,30] this will be discussed in Chapter 11. Estrogens in these pills can cause benign liver growths as well, which can bleed extensively and cause problems related to bleeding.

Daughters of women who received DES (diethylstilbestrol) therapy during pregnancy have developed cancer of the cervix and vagina. Sons of mothers who took DES are at higher risk of developing cancer of the testicles because DES causes urinary tract abnormalities including undescended testicles, which, if not corrected surgically before age 6, can develop into cancer of the testicles.[31] Furthermore, women exposed to these same synthetic estrogens in adult life have a higher risk of developing cancer of the cells that line the inside of the uterus (endometrial cancer). Male hormones can predispose to both benign and malignant liver tumors.

Obesity is directly correlated with breast cancer[32,33,34,35] and endometrial cancer.[36] This subject will be discussed in Chapter 8.

Fibrocystic breast disease, a benign disease which affects 50 percent of all women sometime during their lives, probably represents a hormone imbalance. If a woman has had the disease over many years, she is at an increased risk of developing breast cancer.[37,38] Recently, as will be discussed in Chapter 6, fibrocystic breast disease has appeared to respond to vitamin E therapy.

SEXUAL-SOCIAL RISK FACTORS

Cancer of the female cervix is associated with an early age of sexual intercourse and with multiple male sexual partners. The earlier the age of starting sexual intercourse, and the greater the number of male partners a female has, the higher is her risk of getting cancer of the cervix. Uncircumcised male partners may also contribute to the risk of developing cervical cancer of the female.

Cancer of the penis is a very rare disease in the United States. There is almost universal agreement that one primary risk factor is responsible for this cancer. The risk factor is poor hygiene, especially in the uncircumcised person. Secretion and different organisms retained under the foreskin produce irritation and infection which are thought to predispose to cancer cellular changes.[39]

There is an epidemic outbreak of Kaposi's sarcoma in sexually active male homosexuals.[40,41,42] Kaposi's sarcoma is a cancer of the skin, mucous membranes, and lymph nodes. Those affected have an acquired immuno-deficiency syndrome (AIDS).

Sexually active male homosexuals in good health can have a normal or an abnormal immune system. Many with an abnormal immune system appear quite healthy. Some with a malfunctioning immune system have had Kaposi's sarcoma and/or fatal or life-threatening infections caused by Pneumocystis carinii.[43,44]

The immune impairment (AIDS) seen in sexually active male homosexuals has been reported as having several causes. The first is amyl nitrite, a drug which is currently in vogue as a sexual stimulant. This drug, as well as a closely related compound, isobutyl nitrite, is openly used in homosexual bars and baths. Amyl nitrite produces a profound impairment of the immune system, especially the T lymphocytes.[45] Second, male homosexuals experience repeated infections with a virus called cytomegalovirus (CMV), which has been found in cancer cells of Kaposi's sarcoma. CMV together with an abnormal immune system predispose to Kaposi's sarcoma. Third, immunological abnormalities are seen more often in homosexuals who have many sexual partners than in those who have only one partner.[46] Most, if not all, homosexuals who have Kaposi's sarcoma have had many sexual partners.

Hence, sexually active male homosexuals who use amyl nitrite and/or have many sexual partners are at risk for Kaposi's sarcoma. In addition to Kaposi's sarcoma, male homosexuality is a risk factor for two other cancers: cancer of the anus[47] and cancer of the tongue.

VIRAL RISK FACTORS

Viruses have been shown to directly cause cancer in fish, birds, frogs, and almost every mammal. Over one hundred viruses capable of causing cancer have been identified. Thus far, no cancer in man has been proved to be caused by a virus. There are some cancers in man that are highly *suspected* of being caused by a virus, but this has not been proven. Genetic parts of viruses have been found in certain human cancer cells. It may eventually be proven that at least some human cancers are caused by certain viruses.

RADIATION RISK FACTORS

Studies in humans show that the more radiation a person gets, the higher the risk of developing cancer, especially if the radiation exposure is to bone marrow, where the blood cells are made. People who received radiation to shrink enlarged tonsils or to treat acne have a higher risk of developing cancer of the thyroid and parathyroid glands located in the neck. Survivors of the bombings of Hiroshima and Nagasaki have had an increased incidence of leukemia, lymphoma, Hodgkin's disease, multiple myeloma, and other cancers. People who used to paint radium on wristwatch dials have a high incidence of osteogenic sarcoma, a bone cancer. Chronic exposure to sunlight (ultraviolet light) in fair-skinned people who easily sunburn will lead to a higher rate of skin cancer.

Women with tuberculosis who received many chest X-rays to follow the progress of treatment had an increased incidence of breast cancer with as little as 17.0-rad total dose. A rad is a defined amount of energy (100 ergs) absorbed by a certain amount of body tissue (cubic centimeter). To put things into perspective, one chest X-ray using modern equipment delivers about 0.14 rad. Riding in an airplane at 35,000 feet for six hours exposes a person to 0.01 rad.

A recent study by Matanoski published in the *Proceedings of the 1980 International Conference on Cancer* indicates that radiologists, besides their well-known increased risk for developing cancer, may also have a 30 percent increased risk of death from cardiovascular disease and stroke due to radiation exposure. Workers in many industries are chronically exposed to low-dose radiation and hence may be at risk for heart disease and cancer. We may therefore have to reexamine standards for acceptable radiation levels in industry.

In the following chapters we will review nutritional risk factors, other risk factors that can lead to the development of cancer, and ways that the risk factors can be modified.

AIR AND WATER POLLUTION

Air pollution in cities may be a risk factor for cancer, especially lung cancer, because of the following. More people in cities smoke cigarettes than in rural areas. Carcinogens derived from car emissions, industrial activity, burning of solid wastes and fuels remain in the air from four to forty days and thereby travel long distances.[48] And asbestos, a potent carcinogen, can also be found airborne in cities.

Our drinking water contains a number of carcinogens, including asbestos, arsenic, metals, and synthetic organic compounds.[49,50] Asbestos and nitrates are associated with gastrointestinal cancers; arsenic is associated with skin cancer; and, synthetic organic chemicals are associated with cancers of the gastrointestinal tract and urinary bladder.

As with many carcinogens, the time between exposure to the carcinogen and actual development of cancer may be quite long. Hence, the cause of a cancer initiated by trace amounts of either airborne or waterborne carcinogens years before may be attributed to an unrelated or unknown cause at time of diagnosis. We are able to detect many carcinogens in our environment, but many others exist in low concentrations. These environmental carcinogens may themselves develop cancers or they may interact with other risk factors to initiate, or promote, cancers. Therefore, our environment, a risk factor for cancer, must be modified by keeping it clean.

TWO

The Body's Defenses

3

The Backbone of Nutrition: Proteins, Carbohydrates, and Lipids

NUTRITION is a complex subject, confusing to the public and to some physicians as well. Since roughly half of all cancers are related to nutritional factors, it is important to understand how diet exerts an effect on the development of cancer.

Food may contain carcinogens (chemicals which can cause cancer) either as natural components of the food or in the form of additives. Carcinogens may be inhaled or may exist in our drinking water. Carcinogens may be present in food that is spoiled (by bacteria, fungus, or chemicals), improperly washed, or contaminated with industrial pollutants. Processing or cooking may activate existing carcinogens in foods. Food products may contain nitrite preservatives, which can form an extremely potent carcinogen, nitrosamine. Intestinal bacteria may be altered by diets high in animal fat and cholesterol, and these altered types of bacteria may activate or produce carcinogens from the ingested food or bile acids. If a person is undernourished with respect to protein, carbohydrates, vitamins, or minerals, he will be particularly susceptible to the effects of carcinogens because his immune system will be impaired. Obesity is a risk factor for many cancers and is associated with several women's cancers. People who develop heart disease have many of these same dietary risk factors in common; this will be discussed in Chapter 13. Nutritional deficiencies can directly cause damage to genetic material and then repair it abnormally, which may lead to the development of cancer. Furthermore food, drugs, and hormones (especially estrogens) that we ingest for various reasons may alter body tissues in such a way to predispose the tissue to cancer development. If all these nutritional risk factors can be recognized, then preventive measures can be taken to avoid, eliminate, or at least reduce them. But first, let's review the three main components that make up the backbone of nutrition.

PROTEINS

Proteins are extremely important. Every cell in the body is partly composed of proteins. Each cell is constantly exposed to wear and tear and eventually dies, only to be replaced by another cell. Proteins contribute about 10 to 15 percent of our total energy needs. Enzymes, which are proteins, help most of the body's chemical reactions to proceed quickly. Some very important hormones which are made in the body are proteins as well. In addition, the transport system of the blood is composed of proteins which act as vehicles to carry necessary substances to all parts of the body. Therefore a constant supply of proteins is required so that the body can build tissues and function properly. Our only source of proteins is from the food we eat. Proteins are complex structures consisting of amino acids, some of which cannot be made by the body at all and therefore must be supplied exclusively by the diet. (These include valine, leucine, isoleucine, threonine, lysine, phenyl alanine, tryptophan, methionine, and histidine.) When proteins are eaten, they are broken down into amino acids in the stomach by digesting enzymes and then used by the body to build whatever proteins are needed.

Children and adolescents tend to need more protein than adults, but the amount required varies from one individual to another. A person suffering from burns, bedsores, or other open wounds loses a great deal of protein from these sites. This loss has a deleterious effect because protein is needed to heal wounds in addition to its other functions. An active athlete needs slightly more protein per day than a normally active person because he loses protein through his sweat glands.[1] A pregnant woman also requires more protein than a nonpregnant woman.

A healthy man weighing 140 pounds requires about 28 grams of protein per day, equivalent to about 100 to 115 calories. The source of protein does not have to be from animal meat, a fact that is aptly demonstrated by pure vegetarians who are active and have normal life spans. Seventh-Day Adventists, a religious group composed of many pure vegetarians, have a very low incidence of cancer and heart disease compared to nonvegetarians.

Some sources of proteins are much better than others. Table I lists food sources and percent of usable energy derived from them.[2]

Protein deficiency. Kwashiorkor is an extreme example of protein deficiency which occurs in 1- to 3-year-old children; it was first described by T. Williams in West Africa in 1933. The patient is weak, is emotionally upset, has no appetite, growth is retarded, and there is considerable swelling all over the body. Victims also frequently have vitamin deficiencies and anemia. Another syndrome, called nutritional marasmus, results from a very low intake of all nutrients, including protein. This disorder commonly affects infants during their first year of life and is comparable with starvation in adults.

Table I

Food Source	% Energy
Sweet potatoes	4
Rice	8
Wheat flour	13
Peanuts	19
Cow's milk (3.5% fat)	22
Beans and peas	26
Beef	38
Cow's milk (skimmed)	40
Soybeans	45
Fish	62

CARBOHYDRATES

Carbohydrates provide most of the energy in almost all human diets. They account for 90 percent of poor people's energy needs (poor people consume more junk foods which have a great deal of simple carbohydrates) and 40 percent of affluent people's energy needs. Carbohydrates have an advantage over fats in that they contain less than half the number of calories per ounce. Food carbohydrates consist of complex polysaccharides, starch, glycogen, sucrose, and lactose. Green plants use sunlight to make carbohydrates from carbon dioxide and water. Man has always been able to seek out and grow seeds, fruits, and roots that have concentrated supplies of carbohydrates. Unlike ruminants such as cows, which cannot conserve vegetable foods (cows eat what is available; humans can grow and then store vegetables), humans have been successful in selecting and growing carbohydrate foodstuffs like cereal grain. Complex carbohydrates such as beans, peas, nuts, fruits, vegetables, and whole-grain breads and cereals not only provide calories and essential nutrients but also increase dietary fiber. Dietary fiber (such as lettuce), if eaten daily, can absorb some gastrointestinal carcinogens, increase stool weight, and induce bowel movements daily—all of which decrease the risk of colon cancer. There are some saccharides in certain plants that may be eaten but cannot be digested or absorbed. Our intestinal bacteria can feed on these and produce great amounts of gas as a by-product.

Starch, a complex polysaccharide, is made up of glucose. When ingested, it is broken down into disaccharide and other components that are then further broken down into single glucose units by special enzymes. Cellulose is another polysaccharide found in plants that cannot be digested; it provides most of the roughage in human diets.

Eighty percent of the carbohydrate absorbed from the intestine is in the form of the simple sugar glucose. The main role of glucose is to provide energy for immediate needs. The unused excess glucose is taken to the liver and a small amount is resynthesized into glycogen. Glycogen accumulates in red muscle and is used for its energy. During exertion glycogen is broken down in the muscle for energy use and lactic acid builds up as a waste product. This acid causes the pain perceived in muscles during intensive exercise. Most unused glucose is converted into fat and stored in fat cells which are called adipose tissue. The larger the fat cell, the quicker is the conversion of glucose into fat.[3] In people who are obese, only the size of the fat cells is increased, not the number. The number of fat cells in a person is determined by about age 2 and from then on remains constant. Hence it is important to keep a child 2 years old or under from becoming obese.

When a person ingests carbohydrates, the hormone insulin is released from the pancreas to help utilize the glucose molecules. Obviously the more times you eat carbohydrates in a day the more often the pancreas has to work. There are persons whose insulin is released later than normal and/or over a prolonged time. Insulin in these situations results in a low blood sugar after even a moderate ingestion of carbohydrate.

Diabetes mellitus is a constellation of signs and symptoms which are the result of high blood sugar due to defective insulin release from the pancreas. There is evidence to implicate a number of causes of diabetes: hereditary factors, obesity, chronic alcoholism (which causes pancreatic disease), and a virus. Contrary to a popular old wives' tale, too much sugar in the diet probably does not cause diabetes mellitus.

Carbohydrates available to us in processed foods in the United States are generally depleted of vitamins, minerals, and fiber. (Processing food, per se, can deplete it of vitamins, minerals, and fiber.) You can, however, supplement the diet with vitamins and minerals.

LIPIDS

The word "lipid" is the biochemical term to denote what is commonly called fat. Lipids are very important chemical substances; they include cholesterol, triglycerides, fatty acids, phospholipids, and sterols. Lipids provide a concentrated source of energy, delay the emptying of the stomach, stimulate the gall bladder to empty its contents, and provide the materials for the absorption of fat-soluble vitamins and other dietary substances. Lipids are by far the most important form of storage fuel we have, and they also act as insulation for the body.

Other functions and processes that lipids participate in are much more complex than those of either proteins or carbohydrates. Lipids provide the structure of the brain and all nerve tissue, and they are the major components of all cell membranes and membranes of structures inside cells. As fatty acids and cholesterol esters they store energy in adipose tissue. When energy is needed, free fatty acids are released by the action of stress or epinephrine (adrenaline).

The body can make lipids from carbohydrates and amino acids if enough fats are not supplied from the diet. This is usually not the case in the American diet, though.

Adipose tissue is composed of between 60 and 90 percent

triglycerides. Triglycerides are one major group in the lipid family. The normal serum (blood) level of triglycerides ranges from 10 to 150 mg/ml. Triglycerides and cholesterol, another lipid, are of major clinical significance in the development of heart and vascular disease. Lipoproteins (proteins coupled to lipids) are important in relation to heart disease, also. The following terms are frequently used when discussing the causes of heart disease, colon cancer, and breast cancer: *Chylomicrons* are large particles in which cholesterol and other lipids in the diet are transported from the intestine into the blood. *Very low density lipoproteins* (VLDL) are proteins in the blood that transport trigylcerides that are made in the body. VLDL are broken down to *low-density lipoproteins* (LDL), which are considered by some to cause atherosclerosis. *High-density lipoproteins* (HDL) contain cholesterol and aid in the chemical reaction that modifies cholesterol. HDL is the most important of these proteins for our discussion because it correlates fairly well with heart disease.

For an analogy of HDL's importance and function, consider that each HDL is a street bus, and a blood vessel is a street, and each cholesterol molecule is a person. Now consider that there is only one bus (one HDL) to pick up one hundred people (one hundred cholesterols) along the street. Well, obviously not all the people can be transported by the bus and many people have to stay in the street. In this situation with only one HDL, the cholesterol molecules which were not picked up get embedded in the blood vessel and start to form narrowing and hardening of the artery—atherosclerosis is the medical term. If there are two buses (two HDLs), then more people (cholesterol) can be transported and fewer are left behind to stay in the street (get embedded in the artery). If four buses are available, all the people can be transported and none are left behind (all the cholesterol is transported and none embeds into arteries). Cholesterol is crucial to the development and progression of atherosclerosis. The level of HDL is important only if the cholesterol level is high. With very high cholesterol (people), one would want to try to raise the HDL level (buses). The HDL protein can be raised by vigorous exercise, by administering small amounts of alcohol (details in Chapter 13), and by decreasing substantially the total intake of cholesterol in one's diet.

Cholesterol exists in all animal cells. Everyone requires cholesterol in correct amounts for good health, but too much can lead to the development of heart and blood vessel disease. It is a precursor substance needed for the manufacture of sex hormones and some adrenal hormones which regulate many phases of salt, sugar, protein, and fat metabolism in the body. Part of the cholesterol in your body comes from food of animal origin, and part is made in your body. Cholesterol content is very high in many foods such as eggs, milk products, and organ meats (liver, etc.). It is moderately high in shellfish.

The normal cholesterol range is from 150 to 250 mg/ml. One third of the U.S. male population 25 years old and older have serum cholesterols over 250 mg/ml and are at risk of developing coronary heart disease and vascular disease. Table I in Chapter 16 provides a comprehensive list of foods and their cholesterol contents. There is no cholesterol in foods of plant origin—fruits, vegetables, grains, cereals, and nuts.

Fatty acids are part of the lipid family also. There are three types: First there are the saturated fatty acids, which consist predominately of saturated fats hardened at room temperatures. Saturated fats tend to raise the blood cholesterol level and should be restricted or totally eliminated from your diet. Most Americans eat foods which are high in saturated fats and high in cholesterol and therefore tend to have high cholesterol levels. People who eat high-cholesterol, high-saturated-fat foods have a greater risk of having heart attacks than people who eat low-fat, low-cholesterol diets. Eating extra cholesterol and saturated fat increases blood cholesterol levels in most people, but there are wide variations among individuals, related to heredity and to how the person uses cholesterol. It appears that some people can eat diets which are high in saturated fats and cholesterol and still maintain normal blood levels of cholesterol, while other people cannot. Unfortunately, some people have high blood cholesterol levels even though they eat low-fat, low-cholesterol foods.

Saturated animal fats are found in beef, lamb, pork, and ham; in butter, cream, and whole milk; and in cheeses made from cream and whole milk. Saturated vegetable fats are found in many hydrogenated and solid shortenings; and in coconut oil, cocoa butter, and palm oil (used in commercially prepared cookies, pie fillings, and nondairy milk and cream substitutes).

The other two groups of fatty acids are the unsaturated fats, with a single unsaturated site, and the polyunsaturated fats, which have two or more unsaturated sites in the fat chain. An unsaturated site does not have hydrogen in it; if enough hydrogen were added, the fat would then become saturated or hydrogenated. Fats with a high proportion of unsaturated fat sites are usually liquid at room temperatures (cod liver oil, olive oil, whale oil). There is only one essential fatty acid: arachidonic acid. This can easily be made in the body from linoleic acid, which is widespread in nature. In reality, a deficiency of fatty acids is very rare in humans.

Polyunsaturated fats are liquid oils of vegetable origin. The following oils are high in polyunsaturated fats and are recommended to be used sparingly in your diet: corn, cottonseed, safflower, sesame seed, soybean, and sunflower seed. These lower the blood cholesterol level by eliminating newly formed excess cholesterol. Peanut oil and olive oil are vegetable oils, but they are low in polyunsaturated fats. Don't substitute these two for the above vegetable oils, but you can use them for flavoring foods. Be careful to read the labels on salad dressings, cooking fats, and margarines: they should contain polyunsaturated vegetable oils for their cholesterol-lowering effect. The idea is to make sure that the fat you do eat is polyunsaturated.

And even this should be kept to a severe minimum because, as you will read in Chapter 5, polyunsaturated fats can be attacked chemically and free radicals can be created. These free radicals can damage cells and lead to the development of cancer. There are, however, antiradical agents like vitamin E, vitamin C, and selenium that we can take daily to aid in our defense.

4

Nutrition, Immunity, and Cancer

POOR populations around the world who are malnourished are more susceptible to infection than those who receive adequate nutrition. Investigators studying the relationship between the immune system and nutrition have found that nutrition affects immunity[1] and also affects the development of cancer[2,3] either directly or indirectly via the immune system.

The immune system is a complex interaction of blood cells, proteins, and processes which protects people from infections, foreign substances, and cancer cells which spontaneously develop in the body.

White blood cells and antibodies are two major armies of the immune system. These armies arise separately but are related and dependent upon each other for their development and maturity. The lymphocyte, a specific type of white blood cell, is the main cell involved in cellular immunity. There are not many lymphocytes in the blood—only about 15 to 20 percent of all white cells. The lymphocyte population is divided into two large groups, based on particular markings on the outer surface membrane covering of the cell.

T lymphocytes, or T cells, are one group of lymphocytes. They are derived from or are under the influence of the *t*hymus, which is an organ in the neck and front part of the chest that is functionally active in early childhood. T cells are responsible for a person's defense against cancer, fungus, certain bacteria (intracellular), some viruses, transplant rejections, and delayed skin reactions (tuberculosis skin test). T cells are further divided into several subpopulations: helper T cells and suppressor T cells, those which either help or hinder normal immune cellular function.

Proteins called antibodies or immunoglobulins are produced by the other major group of lymphocytes, the B lymphocytes, or B cells. B cells may have their origin in the *b*one marrow, from which they derive their designation. Antibodies are formed by the B cell in response to a foreign substance introduced into the body. For example, when a person is given a vaccine against polio, antibodies to this foreign substance are made by the B cells. If the polio virus enters the body in an infectious state after a person has been vaccinated, the previously formed antibody, which is circulating in the blood, will attach to this foreign intruder and dispose of it with the help of killing white blood cells or other proteins called complement proteins or a combination of both. The same process of antibody production is initiated by some cancer cells. Killing white blood cells or complement proteins, when activated by an antibody, destroy a foreign-appearing cell by making holes in the foreign cell's membrane, thereby allowing water to rush in and explode the cell. In 1980 we showed how a white blood cell kills a foreign cancerlike cell. Figure 2 shows a white blood cell (center) killing several cancerlike cells. Notice that the white blood cell extends feetlike processes which aid in killing the targets.[4]

Phagocytes are another group of white blood cells which reside in the blood and body's tissues and are part of a person's defenses against foreign invaders. These also act as policemen to recognize and dispose of abnormal cancer cells and other foreign substances. Phagocytes can perform this task alone or can recruit antibodies and complement proteins to aid in the disposal.

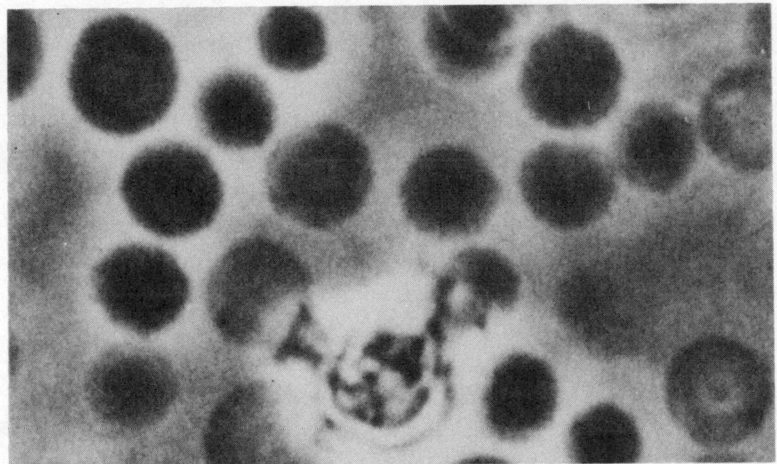

Figure 2. White blood cell (center) killing several cancerlike cells. Notice that the white blood cell extends feetlike processes which aid in killing the targets.

IMMUNOLOGY AND CANCER

The immune system is extremely intricate and finely tuned. If any one aspect of the system malfunctions because of poor nutrition, or is destroyed, the person may become susceptible to cancer and foreign microbial invaders. The white blood cell army and the antibody army must be functioning perfectly to destroy any cancer cell or foreign invader from gaining a foothold in your body.

The major histocompatibility complex is part of the genetic makeup of a person and is another component of the immune system, acting as a commander of the white blood cell and antibody armies. This complex allows a person to recognize all parts of his body as his own so that the immune system does not destroy its own body. At the same time, it can recognize a substance or tissue (histo-) as not belonging to its body and subsequently take the necessary steps to destroy it. The histocompatibility complex is responsible for rejection of transplanted organs such as kidneys and hearts. If the histocompatibility complex is not working properly, a virus capable of converting normal cells to cancer cells may enter the body and not get destroyed because the immune system did not recognize it as foreign. The virus, if not destroyed, will convert normal cells to cancer cells (called transformation) and the cancer will grow and grow and kill the person.

In 1970 F. M. Burnet introduced the concept of immunosurveillance, which states that killer cells of the immune system watch, or keep a surveillance, on all cells in the body and immediately destroy any cells that start to have a malignant or cancerous potential.[5] There is a lot of evidence to support this concept. The most clear-cut and convincing evidence comes from observations of patients with a suppressed immune system, caused by drugs or radiation or an inherited disorder. Patients with inherited immunodeficiencies—whose immune system does not function normally from birth or whose immune system acquires a malfunction later in life—have one hundred times more deaths due to cancer than the expected cancer death rate in the normal population.[6,7] Kidney transplant patients, who receive drugs to suppress the immune system's ability to reject the new kidney, also have a higher rate of cancer than would be expected.[8,9] The cancers most frequently seen in these cases are the lymphomas and epithelial cancers; however, all other types of cancers have been reported as well.

The immune system is relatively immature in infancy, and then gets very lazy and does not function well in old age. These two times of life have the highest incidence of lymphocytic leukemia. Other immune-deficiency states which can lead to cancer are seen with malaria, acute viral infections, and malnutrition.

NUTRITION AND THE IMMUNE SYSTEM

Nutritional deficiencies decrease a person's capacity to resist infection and its consequences and decrease the capability of the immune system. In old age, there is a decrease in skin hypersensitivity reactions, a decreased number of T cells, and impairment of some phagocytic functions. Surveys of the population have discovered nutritional deficiencies in senior citizens, which also lead to impairment of the immune system. It is possible that the gradual impairment of the immune system associated with aging may in fact be due to one or more nutrient deficiencies. Poor nutrition adversely affects all components of the immune system including T cell function, other cellular related killing, the ability of B cells to make antibodies, the complement proteins, and phagocytic function. When several of these functions or processes are impaired, the ability of the entire immune system to keep a watchful eye for and dispose of cancer cells, abnormal cells, or foreign substances is also markedly impaired.

Protein deficiency affects all the organs in the body. Digestive enzymes are reduced and absorption of nutrients is impaired. With severe chronic protein deficiency the heart muscle dwindles away. The immune system is also severely affected. In diets that are only moderately deficient in protein, phagocytes and T cells are reduced in number,[10] and their ability to kill cancer and other abnormal cells is impaired.[11] The amount of antibody is slightly reduced as well as the speed with which it attaches to an "enemy."[12] The complement proteins also have impaired function in this state. Hence, a person who is not consuming the proper amount of protein will have a malfunctioning immune system which will not be able to deal effectively with cancer cells or infection.

The immune system is affected by either hypoglycemia (low blood sugar) or hyperglycemia, as in diabetes mellitus. C. J.

Van Oss has found that phagocytic function in humans is impaired if the blood sugar level is very low.[13] Much more work has been done concerning the function of the immune system in diabetes. The number of T and B cells is normal in diabetes, but their functions are impaired: phagocytic function as well as cellular killing.[14,15] The degree of impairment correlates very well with the fasting blood sugar level and then improves when the sugar level becomes normal.

Lipids have a real impact on the immune system. Cholesterol oleate and ethyl palmitate impair the initiation of antibody production, probably because these lipids do not allow the immune system to recognize the foreign substance.[16] E. A. Santiago-Delpin and J. Szepsenwol wanted to know what effects lipids had on T lymphocytes.[17] They first grafted pieces of skin from one mouse to another dissimilar genetic mouse and found that the grafted skin was rejected in a very short time. They then fed the recipient mouse a high-fat diet and found that it accepted the graft for a very prolonged time, indicating that the high-fat diet impaired the ability of the animal to reject the foreign graft. The T cell is involved in this kind of rejection as well as in cancer cell rejection, and its ability to function is impaired if one eats a high-fat diet. In other experiments, phagocytosis was studied. Another saturated fat, methyl palmitate, was found to markedly impair phagocytosis for at least seventy-two hours after a single injection of this fat.[18] There is great controversy and discrepancy among experiments dealing with polyunsaturated fats and their effect on the immune system. Some investigators report that a diet deficient in polyunsaturated fats has good effects on the immune system,[19] and others report that polyunsaturated fats are less beneficial.[20] In all these studies, it must be kept in mind that the significance of the results is unclear because large amounts of lipids were used. It has not been determined whether physiological doses of the same lipids have similar effects on the immune system as do these large amounts of lipids.

Different people infected by the Epstein-Barr virus may express entirely different diseases. This is the result of each person's varying degree of impairment of the immune system, which is related in part to the nutritional status of that individual. Epstein-Barr virus is implicated in causing a relatively benign disease, infectious mononucleosis; a slow-growing cancer, nasopharyngeal cancer; and a rapidly growing, usually fatal, cancer, Burkitt's lymphoma; as well as other diseases. Why does one person's immune system permit infectious mononucleosis to develop and another person's immune system permit a fatal cancer to develop? The answer is very complex and not well defined at all, but nutritional status is a factor. The better the nutritional status, the better the immune system, and the better off the person will be.

5

Free Radicals

FREE radicals are made in our bodies and, if not destroyed, can lead to the development of cancer. By definition, free radicals are chemical substances which contain an odd number of electrons. Every atom has a nucleus and a certain number of electrons which orbit around the nucleus. This setup is very much like our solar system, with the sun in the middle and all the planets orbiting around the sun. The nucleus has a positive charge, and the electrons have a negative charge. The negative charges of electrons balance out the positive charge of the nucleus to give an overall charge of zero. Hence, the energy of a single atom is very stable at zero. When high energy in any form (light, radiation, etc.) hits an atom, an electron is kicked out of orbit. All of the energy that forced the electron out of orbit is transferred directly to the electron, making it highly energetic and unstable. Because it is so unstable, this electron quickly seeks *another* atom to reside in. This excited high-energy electron transfers very high energy to the new atom, which then becomes extremely unstable because of the newly acquired high energy. (An analogy to this state is a nine-month-old child who has a great deal of energy but is extremely unstable if unattended.) This excited high-energy atom with its extra electron is called a radical. A radical is unstable and must get rid of all the extra energy for the atom to once again become stable, and hence the radical transfers its energy to nearby substances. (All these reactions take place within a fraction of a second.) When radicals are made in the body, the high energy is transferred to body tissues and causes extreme damage to them. If not counteracted, this process can lead to the development of cancer of the tissue affected by the radical.

FORMATION OF RADICALS

Oxygen

There are many processes in the body which initiate destructive radical reactions. Oxygen is crucial to us because it is required for all animal life. In certain instances, however, oxygen can be activated or split with high energy into very potent damaging radicals (superoxide) or a high-energy, unstable nonradical called singlet oxygen. Singlet oxygen has extremely high energy and is very unstable and thus is very destructive to normal body tissues and cells.

Oxygen radicals can be both beneficial and harmful to us at different times under different circumstances. It is a beneficial reaction when a phagocyte kills an invading bacteria.[1] This destruction is accomplished by oxygen radicals, which are made by the phagocyte when a foreign substance like a bacteria is ingested and taken inside the phagocyte. On the other hand, oxygen radicals can produce hydroperoxides, which are chemicals that form more radicals and damage cell membranes, thereby altering the cell's function.[2] This can lead to the development of cancer. Singlet oxygen, a very-high-energy form of oxygen, has a shorter life than an oxygen radical but damages cells and tissues much more quickly. Not only does singlet oxygen have the potential of causing cancer by itself but it also activates carcinogens.

Lipids

A second major process which initiates destructive radicals involves polyunsaturated fatty acids. As you recall, saturated fats were to be avoided and polyunsaturated fats were to be consumed only moderately. The reason for recommending minimal intake of polyunsaturated fats is that when oxygen or enzymes react with polyunsaturated fats to release their energy, a free radical is made. This free radical reacts with another polyunsaturated fat to produce a lot of hydroperoxide.[3,4] The more unsaturated the fat is, the more hydroperoxides are made. And hydroperoxides produce more radicals, damage cell membranes, and can lead to the development of cancer.

Metals

Certain metal accumulations in the body can also initiate free radical formation by activating oxygen. Iron overload is one example of a metal that can form extremely potent hydroxyl radicals.

Radiation

Ionizing radiation produces radicals and electrons which react to yield many different kinds of free radicals. Background radiation in the atmosphere at sea level probably does not produce free radicals in the body, however.[5] Radicals produced in the body and by pollutants are much more important than those caused by radiation unless, of course, a person is receiving large doses of radiation for the treatment of a disease. At high levels of radiation, hydroperoxides are produced in addition to all the other free radicals.[6]

Light from the Sun—Photolysis

All life on earth requires the sun's energy. But sunlight also has a harmful effect on our skin. Excessive sunlight can cause several types of skin cancer. Since millions of people enjoy getting a dark suntan, it is important to review this topic. There is an increasing number of chemicals which we eat or are exposed to that make our skin more sensitive to the damaging effects of sunlight. Ultraviolet light inhibits genetic material (DNA) synthesis, protein synthesis, interrupts normal cell replication, and causes skin cancer. Free radical formation by ultraviolet light may be involved in producing all these effects on the skin's cells. Ultraviolet light has been shown to produce free radicals in skin cells in the test tube,[7] and free radicals are probably responsible for the damaging effects on the skin, including skin cancer. These light rays represent only 0.1 percent of the total sun's energy that comes to us. Chronic sun exposure in Caucasians directly damages the uppermost skin cells and results in wrinkling, the formation of tiny networks of blood vessels, and discrete small raised bumps on the skin called actinic keratosis (which are precancerous).

Ultraviolet light affects the immune system in several ways. A mild sunburn decreases the function of circulating lymphocytes for as long as twenty-four hours. In animals ultraviolet light suppresses the entire immune system so much that skin tumors grow uninhibited.

A fad that has swept the country in the past several years is suntanning booths which offer "year-round" suntans at a minimum charge. The ultraviolet light used in many of these booths is of higher energy (wavelengths of 270 to 350) than the ultraviolet light that we receive when we sunbathe naturally. This higher-energy ultraviolet light is worse for the skin than the light ordinarily received from the sun.

Skin cancers in Caucasians occur most often in those who work out of doors and in those who live in areas with intensive sunlight most of the year (the tropics). Skin cancers are very rare in black people or other people with deeply pigmented skin. Their dark skin protects them against ultraviolet-light damage. The Scottish and Irish, who are the lightest-complexioned peoples, have the highest incidence of skin cancer if they live in areas of the world with high ultraviolet-light exposure. Skin cancers usually arise in areas of the body that are exposed to the sun, except in blacks, in whom skin cancers occur anywhere on the body when they do occur.

Skin cancer is the most common of all human cancers. There are three main types: basal cell cancer, squamous cell cancer, and melanoma. Squamous cell cancer is directly caused by sun exposure, and about 66 percent of all basal cell skin cancers occur in areas of the body exposed to sunlight. The influence of sunlight on forming melanoma, a very deadly cancer, is not conclusively established, but a number of surveys do suggest that sunlight does develop some melanomas.

F. Urbach and others point out that skin cancers develop with three primary factors.[8] The total sunlight exposure in a lifetime is an important factor for developing skin cancer. The more time you are exposed, the higher is the incidence of cancer (people living in Texas and Australia have more skin cancers than people living in North Dakota and Germany). It has also been found that the total time of exposure at one sitting and the frequency of these sittings (especially at wavelengths 290–320 as in many suntanning booths) increase the risk of developing skin cancer. And finally, there are certain inherited diseases, such as xeroderma pigmentosum, which predispose to developing skin cancer. In addition, people without any apparent diseases are prone to developing skin cancers if they have light eyes and light hair color, fair complexion, poor ability to tan, and get sunburned easily with a repeated history of sunburning.

As was pointed out before, certain chemicals (tars, petroleum products, etc.) can cause skin cancer also. The mechanism of this is not clear, but it may involve free radicals.

What defenses do we have against the harmful and cancer-producing effects of sunlight? We can do many commonsense things to lessen our risk of getting skin cancer. First of all, before sunbathing, use one of the several commercially available sunscreens on areas of your body that will be exposed. Don't stay out in the sun for a prolonged period of time at one sitting. If you work out of doors, wear protective clothing to minimize the chronic prolonged exposure to sunlight. Don't seek a suntan from a suntanning booth, because the rays usually emitted there are more damaging on the whole.

Eat carrots! Carrots contain a chemical substance called carotene. Carotene is one of the most efficient scavengers of singlet high-energy oxygen. Carotene also localizes to the skin cells when eaten and there partially protects the skin cells from light damage. Eating carrots or ingesting carotene in quantities large enough to color the skin slightly orange is well tolerated by the body, but I don't recommend that degree of carotene in the body. Vitamin E works in a similar fashion in stopping high-energy oxygen (singlet oxygen) damage.

Smog

It has been shown by R. E. Zelac et al. that the amount of ozone in smoggy air causes more tissue damage than does background radiation.[9] Ozone reacts with almost every type of molecule in the body to form free radicals which then damage cells. Ozone in normal amounts in the air can even form radicals with polyunsaturated fatty acids.[10] One other component of smog, peroxyacetyl nitrate, can break down and produce singlet oxygen. Again, free radical scavengers or antioxidants will neutralize and inhibit ozone-induced radicals. These include vitamin E, vitamin C, and selenium.

Smog also contains nitrogen dioxides, which like ozone can form free radicals but to a lesser extent. These nitrogen oxides react with unsaturated fats of human cell membranes to form radicals which can damage the membranes. Antioxidants or radical scavengers like vitamin E can protect the membrane against radicals.

The components of smog, tobacco smoking, and other air pollutants can form radicals, especially in the lungs. Lung cancer is the leading cause of cancer deaths and is most common in the heavily industrialized areas of the country.

Alcohol and Carbon Tetrachloride

It is now known that excess alcohol and *certain* chloride-containing compounds (vinyl chloride, chloroprene, carbon tetrachloride) react with some enzymes (specifically microsomal mixed function oxidase system) in the liver to produce free radicals.[11,12] These radicals can then locally damage liver cells and potentiate liver cancer or other deadly liver diseases.

OUR BODY'S DEFENSES AGAINST RADICALS

We know that all life requires oxygen, but sometimes oxygen can produce radicals and high-energy (singlet) oxygen. Because of this, most animals have developed many lines of defense against free radical formation to preserve their very existence and to lessen the chance of abnormal cell (cancer) development.

There are many mechanisms which prevent or decrease the occurrence of radicals and the formation of hydroperoxide and thereby decrease the amount of cell membrane damage. The most obvious one is the protective protein coat that lines the surface of the cell membrane. This protective coat prevents oxygen from directly reacting with lipids in the membrane, which otherwise would produce many free radicals. In this situation the protein coat is called an antioxidant, a substance which works against (anti-) oxidation (the process in which oxygen reacts with another chemical) and thereby prevents the harmful effects of oxygen on tissue via radical formation.

A second mechanism involves protective enzymes which float around in all cell membranes. These are another group of antioxidants; they prevent radical formation and also convert existing hydroperoxyl radicals into stable oxygen and hydrogen peroxide. They eliminate the danger of radicals and prevent

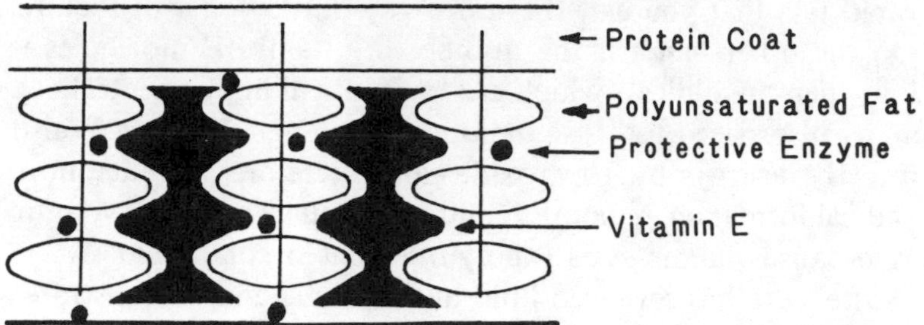

Figure 3. Simplified membrane structure

radical damage to the cell membrane. These protective enzymes are small proteins which swim in the membrane fluid around polyunsaturated fats and hence are in close proximity to them. They include superoxide dismutase,[13] catalase,[14] and selenium-containing glutathione peroxidase.[15] Figure 3 represents a gross simplification of the cell membrane. The enzymes are denoted by a dark dot. Glutathione peroxidase, which is the main enzyme that destroys hydroperoxides, contains the metal selenium in very small amounts. Without selenium, glutathione peroxidase will not function properly. So if there is a slight dietary deficiency in selenium, glutathione peroxidase will not destroy hydroperoxides and a great deal of tissue damage will result from radical formation.

There is a very narrow but equal space between polyunsaturated fat molecules. One vitamin E molecule just fits snugly between them. This location and closeness to the polyunsaturated fats is extremely important. Vitamin E is also an antioxidant and is the third mechanism which inhibits radical formation and thereby prevents their destructive damage. Vitamin E competes with the polyunsaturated fat for free radicals that are formed when polyunsaturated fats react with oxygen. This means that if there are more vitamin E molecules than polyunsaturated fat molecules, the radicals will be taken out of the system and neutralized by vitamin E. The more polyunsaturated fats that you eat, the more vitamin E you will require. On the other hand, if the number of vitamin E molecules is low, then the radicals which are formed will not be neutralized and will proceed to cause membrane damage. Vitamin E also directly destroys hydroperoxides and therefore prevents more radical formation. Vitamin E and selenium also protect vitamin A because vitamin A is a polyunsaturated compound. W. L. Wattenberg has reviewed lipid antioxidants and demonstrated their role in preventing cancer.[16] The process of aging is also most probably related to hydroperoxide action on lipids. Aging is thought to be due to the process of oxidation.

Free radicals are unstable chemical substances with high energy. Normal enzymes can produce free radicals, which can form more radicals and singlet oxygen (very-high-energy oxygen). Oxygen reacting with lipids to free its stored energy may also produce hydroperoxides. All of these will cause tissue damage and may lead to the development of cancer. The body does have defenses to protect itself against these, including the protective protein coat of the cell membrane, protective enzymes (catalase, superoxide dismutase, and selenium-containing glutathione peroxidase), and vitamin E. In the next chapter, we will investigate the vitamins and minerals and their role in protecting us.

6

Vitamins and Minerals

LIVING cells contain proteins, nucleic acids, carbohydrates, lipids, and certain organic substances that function in very small amounts, called vitamins. It has been known for centuries that many diseases are directly related to diet. Night blindness was cured by eating liver. In the eighteenth century cod liver oil was used to treat rickets. The juice of limes was found to prevent the symptoms of scurvy among British sailors in the late eighteenth century (and from then on, the sailors were known as "limeys"). F. G. Hopkins in England proved in 1912 that animals require certain "accessory factors" in addition to protein, fat, and carbohydrate. In the same year Casimer Funk lessened the symptoms of beriberi among Japanese sailors by giving them an extract of rice husks, which was an amine. He was the first to denote this essential amine as *vitamine* (*vita* means life). Shortly thereafter, a scientist in the United States named E. V. McCollum showed that animals need both water-soluble and fat-soluble vitamins to maintain proper existence. Then it was discovered that bacteria which normally live in our intestines to help with food digestion can produce some of the vitamins that we require.

Vitamins are divided into two groups: those which are soluble in fat and those which are soluble in water. Fat-soluble vitamins are vitamins A, D, E, and K. And those which are soluble in water are thiamine (B_1), riboflavin (B_2), nicotinic acid, pantothenic acid, pyridoxine (B_6), biotin, folic acid, vitamin B_{12}, lipoic acid, and ascorbic acid (C).

Vitamins are essential to life and play a crucial role as helper enzymes in important chemical functions of the body. If there are deficiencies of vitamins, a variety of diseases may occur, and the immune system will not function properly.

Vitamins interact with each other, and a few are toxic in high doses. Some vitamins can be stored for long periods of time, while others have to be supplied on a daily basis. We now know that certain drugs and hormones can produce a gradual vitamin deficiency by interfering with the ways in which vitamins are broken down for use in the body. Vitamins are also needed for normal prenatal development. Vitamins are of great interest because of their interplay among all organ systems of the body, especially the immune system.

What are the proper amounts of vitamins that we should ingest daily? Recently, the 1980 Recommended Dietary Allowances were published by the National Academy of Sciences. Recommended Dietary Allowances (RDAs) are the levels of intake of essential nutrients considered to be adequate to meet the nutritional needs of most healthy people in the United States, as judged by the Committee on Dietary Allowances of the Food and Nutrition Board.

Recommended Dietary Allowances were established in 1943 to be used as a guide for planning and purchasing food supplies for the armed forces. RDAs are recommendations for the average daily amount of nutrients that healthy people should consume over a period of time and are estimated to exceed the requirements of most individuals. The RDAs are revised every five years. Needs for extra nutrients arise from such problems as inherited disorders, infections, cancer, chronic diseases, and the use of some medications. The current RDAs are listed in Table I. Conditions that may require some adjustments in RDAs are:

1. *Stress.* Stress, like overwork and tension, increases the need for some vitamins.

2. *Physical activity.* Any activity or condition that increases sweating and thereby a loss of salt and water, if prolonged, may lead to significant losses of other essential nutrients.

3. *Climate.* Prolonged exposure to high temperatures may reduce activity and energy expenditure and therefore food intake.

4. *Age.* Although there is usually a decrease in physical activity as one gets older, the nutrient needs remain unchanged.

5. *Clinical diseases.* Infections increase the loss of protein and many vitamins and minerals. Cancer requires more vitamins as well. The period of recuperation following illnesses, trauma, burns, and surgical procedures requires extra nutrients.

6. *Pregnancy.* More vitamins and minerals are required during pregnancy and lactation.

7. *Birth control pills.* Women who take birth control pills may need extra vitamin B_1, B_2, B_{12}, folic acid, and maybe as much as five times the normal RDA of vitamin B_6. Low vitamin B_6 may result in symptoms of depression.

8. *Alcohol.* Drinking alcohol may interfere with the availability of vitamin B_1, B_6, and folic acid. Also, people who drink excessively frequently have poor eating habits and therefore have a reduced total vitamin intake.

9. *Smoking.* Smoking can reduce the blood level of vitamin C by as much as 30 percent.

10. *Weight reduction.* People who are trying to lose weight by just reducing the amounts of food normally eaten and totally eliminating some foods may need extra vitamins. If caloric intake is below 1200 calories per day, vitamin and mineral supplementation is needed.

11. *Polyunsaturated fats.* People who consume a large amount of polyunsaturated fats will need an extra amount of antioxidants like vitamin E, C, or selenium for the reasons outlined in the previous chapter.

TABLE I Recommended Daily Dietary Allowances, Revised 1980

Food and Nutrition Board, National Academy of Sciences – National Research Council

Designed for the maintenance of good nutrition of practically all healthy people in the U.S.A.

	Age (years)	Weight (kg)	Weight (lbs)	Height (cm)	Height (in)	Protein (g)	Fat-Soluble Vitamins: Vitamin A (μg R.E.)	Vitamin D (μg)	Vitamin E (mg α T.E.)	Water-Soluble Vitamins: Vitamin C (mg)	Thiamin (mg)	Riboflavin (mg)	Niacin (mg N.E.)	Vitamin B_6 (mg)	Folacin [f] (μg)	Vitamin B_{12} (μg)	Minerals: Calcium (mg)	Phosphorus (mg)	Magnesium (mg)	Iron (mg)	Zinc (mg)	Iodine (μg)
Infants	0.0-0.5	6	13	60	24	kg × 2.2	420	10	3	35	0.3	0.4	6	0.3	30	0.5[g]	360	240	50	10	3	40
	0.5-1.0	9	20	71	28	kg × 2.0	400	10	4	35	0.5	0.6	8	0.6	45	1.5	540	360	70	15	5	50
Children	1-3	13	29	90	35	23	400	10	5	45	0.7	0.8	9	0.9	100	2.0	800	800	150	15	10	70
	4-6	20	44	112	44	30	500	10	6	45	0.9	1.0	11	1.3	200	2.5	800	800	200	10	10	90
	7-10	28	62	132	52	34	700	10	7	45	1.2	1.4	16	1.6	300	3.0	800	800	250	10	10	120
Males	11-14	45	99	157	62	45	1000	10	8	50	1.4	1.6	18	1.8	400	3.0	1200	1200	350	18	15	150
	15-18	66	145	176	69	56	1000	10	10	60	1.4	1.7	18	2.0	400	3.0	1200	1200	400	18	15	150
	19-22	70	154	177	70	56	1000	7.5	10	60	1.5	1.7	19	2.2	400	3.0	800	800	350	10	15	150
	23-50	70	154	178	70	56	1000	5	10	60	1.4	1.6	18	2.2	400	3.0	800	800	350	10	15	150
	51+	70	154	178	70	56	1000	5	10	60	1.2	1.4	16	2.2	400	3.0	800	800	350	10	15	150
Females	11-14	46	101	157	62	46	800	10	8	50	1.1	1.3	15	1.8	400	3.0	1200	1200	300	18	15	150
	15-18	55	120	163	64	46	800	10	8	60	1.1	1.3	14	2.0	400	3.0	1200	1200	300	18	15	150
	19-22	55	120	163	64	44	800	7.5	8	60	1.1	1.3	14	2.0	400	3.0	800	800	300	18	15	150
	23-50	55	120	163	64	44	800	5	8	60	1.0	1.2	13	2.0	400	3.0	800	800	300	18	15	150
	51+	55	120	163	64	44	800	5	8	60	1.0	1.2	13	2.0	400	3.0	800	800	300	10	15	150
Pregnant						+30	+200	+5	+2	+20	+0.4	+0.3	+2	+0.6	+400	+1.0	+400	+400	+150	h	+5	+25
Lactating						+20	+400	+5	+3	+40	+0.5	+0.5	+5	+0.5	+100	+1.0	+400	+400	+150	h	+10	+50

TABLE II Recommended Dietary Allowances, Revised 1980

Food and Nutrition Board, National Academy of Sciences—National Research Council, Washington, D.C.

Estimated Safe and Adequate Daily Dietary Intakes of Selected Vitamins and Minerals

		Vitamins			Trace Elements						Electrolytes		
	Age (years)	Vitamin K (μg)	Biotin (μg)	Pantothenic Acid (mg)	Copper (mg)	Manganese (mg)	Fluoride (mg)	Chromium (mg)	Selenium (mg)	Molybdenum (mg)	Sodium (mg)	Potassium (mg)	Chloride (mg)
Infants	0-0.5	12	35	2	0.5-0.7	0.5-0.7	0.1-0.5	0.01-0.04	0.01-0.04	0.03-0.06	115-350	350-925	275-700
	0.5-1	10-20	50	3	0.7-1.0	0.7-1.0	0.2-1.0	0.02-0.06	0.02-0.06	0.04-0.08	250-750	425-1275	400-1200
Children	1-3	15-30	65	3	1.0-1.5	1.0-1.5	0.5-1.5	0.02-0.08	0.02-0.08	0.05-0.1	325-975	550-1650	500-1500
and	4-6	20-40	85	3-4	1.5-2.0	1.5-2.0	1.0-2.5	0.03-0.12	0.03-0.12	0.06-0.15	450-1350	775-2325	700-2100
Adolescents	7-10	30-60	120	4-5	2.0-2.5	2.0-3.0	1.5-2.5	0.05-0.2	0.05-0.2	0.1-0.3	600-1800	1000-3000	925-2775
	11+	50-100	100-200	4-7	2.0-3.0	2.5-5.0	1.5-2.5	0.05-0.2	0.05-0.2	0.15-0.5	900-2700	1525-4575	1400-4200
Adults		70-140	100-200	4-7	2.0-3.0	2.5-5.0	1.5-4.0	0.05-0.2	0.05-0.2	0.15-0.5	1100-3300	1875-5625	1700-5100

After the food for our American diet has been harvested or slaughtered, it is prepared in large volume for sale and loses much of its nutritional value. You see, the RDAs represent the minimum nutrient levels needed to prevent obvious signs of vitamin deficiencies. These recommended levels are probably *not* the maximum needed for good health. Dr. Linus Pauling, a Nobel laureate, has recently shown in animal studies that the levels of vitamins required to maintain good health varied by 2000 percent from one animal to another of the same species. Dr. Pauling extrapolates from this study that human requirements may vary just as greatly and therefore the RDA for a given food may be one person's exact requirement but not the next person's. Dr. Pauling is quoted by the *Washingtonian* magazine in March 1981 as saying that today's diet does not provide as many vitamins as the diet of two generations ago. Over the past seventy-five years people have increased their consumption of fat by 30 percent and sugar by 50 percent, and have decreased their consumption of vegetables, grains, and fruits by 40 percent. In fact, Dr. Pauling found that 110 raw, natural foods eaten by our grandparents contained two to five times more vitamin A, thiamine (B_1), riboflavin (B_2), and pyridoxine (B_6) than we normally consume today.

It is more difficult to identify a person who is only marginally deficient in vitamins than someone who is obviously deficient. Whereas a person who is grossly deficient in vitamins demonstrates many physical problems and complains about specific symptoms related to the deficiencies, a person with only marginal deficiencies demonstrates no such signs or symptoms and does not appear to be ill. The RDAs were designed for healthy people, and the values recommended may not be adequate for persons developing undetected marginal deficiencies. Recent USDA surveys show that many elderly people have low or deficient levels of folic acid and zinc which have not yet produced symptoms related to these deficiencies.

Outright vitamin deficiencies occur in two groups of people. In the first group, an individual is unable to buy the right kinds of food either because of the expense or because he is not knowledgeable about the proper foods. It is estimated that 25 percent of U.S. households do not have nutritionally balanced diets because people do not know what foods to buy or because vitamins and minerals are lost through cooking. The milling process used to make white flour has been reported to remove twenty-two nutrients from the wheat, including about 90 percent of the vitamin E content. When flour is labeled "enriched," usually only four of these nutrients are replaced: thiamine, riboflavin, niacin, and iron. Sugar refinement also removes most of its vitamins and minerals. Cooked and reheated potatoes are reported to have only 10 percent of the vitamin C content of raw potatoes. The second group consists of people whose nutrient deficiency occurs as the result of a specific disease or a drug or other treatment therapy.

An interesting study done by C. M. Leevy and his collaborators reports on the incidence of low blood levels of vitamins in a randomly selected group of hospitalized patients.[1] Table II shows the vitamin and the percent of people with this deficiency. Only 12 percent of 120 patients had normal vitamin levels (RDA standards); 88 percent had at least one vitamin deficiency. What is even more interesting is that many had more than one vitamin deficiency. In spite of this, 61 percent of the total group of 120 patients were eating what is considered to be a normal American diet!

Specific nutritional deficiencies are also associated with abnormal behavior and learning disabilities. The classic example of this is pellagra, caused by a lack of niacin or certain proteins. Pellagra is characterized by mental derangement (psychosis) and several other symptoms including skin inflammation and diarrhea, and can result in death. A number of vitamins are necessary for normal functioning of the nervous system. For instance: thiamine (B_1) deficiency results in convulsions in in-

Table II

VITAMIN DEFICIENCIES IN HOSPITALIZED PATIENTS

Vitamin	% Deficient	Vitamin	% Deficient
1. Folic acid	45	9. Vitamin C	12
2. Thiamine (B_2)	31	10. Vitamin B_2	10
3. Nicotinic acid	29	11. Biotin	1
4. Pyridoxine (B_6)	27	12. Two deficiencies	38
5. Pantothenic acid	15	13. Three deficiencies	14
6. Vitamin A	13	14. Four deficiencies	6
7. Vitamin E	12	15. Five deficiencies	10
8. Riboflavin (B_2)	12		

fants; pantothenic acid deficiency causes sensory losses in the arms and legs; niacin deficiency causes pellagra; folic acid deficiency causes unclear thinking; vitamin C deficiency causes fatigue; vitamin E deficiency in animals causes brain degeneration; and vitamin A deficiency causes night blindness. Many other medical illnesses may be responsible for these symptoms or behaviors, and all such possibilities must be entertained and excluded by proper workup. However, assuming all other medical illnesses have been ruled out as possible causes, a marginal deficiency of a vitamin may cause subtle early symptoms of these abnormal brain functions.

A person should ingest the proper amount of vitamins and minerals daily, through a well-balanced diet and supplementation, because: (1) vitamins and minerals play a vital role for all organ functions of the body; (2) a marginal deficiency cannot be readily detected in an apparently normal individual; (3) certain vitamins and minerals are antioxidants and help rid the body of free radicals which can lead to the development of cancer; and (4) certain vitamins may have direct anticancer properties.

In the following pages, vitamins and selected minerals will be discussed individually.

Table III

Vitamin	Function	Food Source
Fat soluble		
Vitamin A	Has anticancer properties. Essential for normal immune function. Prevents night blindness. Vital for normal growth, good vision, healthy skin and hair.	Tomatoes, milk, eggs, liver, kidney, fortified margarine, leafy green and yellow vegetables.
Vitamin D	Prevents rickets. Helps body use calcium and phosphorus. Needed for strong teeth and bones.	Milk, tuna, cod liver oil, salmon, egg yolk.
Vitamin E	Is an antioxidant and as such protects against free radicals. Protects against polyunsaturated fats. Vital for red cell function.	Leafy vegetables, wheat germ, whole-grain cereals, vegetable oils.
Vitamin K	Essential for normal blood clotting.	Fresh green leafy vegetables. Beef liver.
Water soluble		
Thiamine (B_1)	Prevents beriberi. Essential for normal function of heart and nervous system.	Bread, flour, enriched cereals, fish, lean meat, liver, milk, pork, poultry, whole-grain cereals.
Riboflavin (B_2)	Helps to degrade drugs and foreign substances. Prevents light-sensitivity of eyes. Builds and maintains body tissues like skin, brain, blood.	Leafy green vegetables, enriched bread and cereals, lean meat, liver, milk, eggs.
Niacin	Prevents pellagra. Helps convert food into energy. Vital for nervous system.	Lean meat, liver, eggs, enriched bread and cereals.

Table III—*Continued*

Vitamin	Function	Food Source
Pantothenic acid	Helps body to use fat, proteins, and carbohydrates.	Virtually all eatable plant and animal food.
Pyridoxine (B_6)	Deficiency leads to decreased antibodies, T cells, and body's ability to reject transplants and cancer cells. Necessary for teeth and gums, red cells, and nervous system.	Vegetables, whole-grain cereals, wheat germ, meat, bananas.
Vitamin B_{12}	Prevents certain anemias. Essential for the nervous system and proper children's growth.	Lean meat, liver, kidney, milk, saltwater fish, oysters.
Folic acid	Prevents certain anemias. Needed for certain functions in intestinal tract.	Fresh green leafy vegetables, lean meats.
Biotin	Deficiency results in anemia and depression. Essential for chemical reactions involving fats, proteins, carbohydrates.	Green vegetables, milk, liver, kidney, egg yolk.
Vitamin C	Antioxidant. Inhibits certain cancers and carcinogens. Deficiency results in decreases in T cell number and phagocytic function. Prevents scurvy. Essential for gums, teeth, bones, body cells, blood vessels.	Citrus fruits and fruit juices, fortified juices, tomatoes, berries, green vegetables, potatoes.

Table III is an easy-reference guide to the vitamins, with a brief description of their function and their food sources.

Fat-Soluble Vitamins

Carotene

Beta-carotene is the chemical precursor that the body uses to make vitamin A. Carrots account for the major source of beta-carotene in North American diets, yellow-green vegetables in Japan, and red palm oil in West Africa. Studies have indicated that people who consume higher than average amounts of beta-carotene have a lower incidence of cancer, and "it is most unlikely that this association will disappear entirely with future observational studies."[1a] It appears that this lower incidence of cancer is attributed to beta-carotene itself, rather than to its conversion for vitamin A. Beta-carotene may inhibit the development of cancer in the following ways: It greatly enhances the immune system. It is a powerful antioxidant, free radical scavenger. Beta-carotene is the most efficient neutralizer of singlet oxygen, the high-energy, destructive molecule (see Chapter 5).

The normal range of human intake of beta-carotene is a few milligrams per day. However, large daily intakes of beta-carotene appear to be harmless; also it does not cause vitamin A toxicity. It is converted to vitamin A only as the body requires it. One or two hundred milligrams per day are regularly prescribed for the treatment of a disease called erythropoietic protoporphyria without causing vitamin A toxicity, liver problems, or any other apparent side effects. The World Health Organization Expert Committee on Food Additives estimated the acceptable daily intake of beta-carotene for a 140-pound adult to be about 350 mg per day.[1b] In several studies, supplemental beta-carotene in the amount of 30 mg per day has been used without harm but has caused yellowing of the skin in a select few persons.

Vitamin A

The new recommended dose for vitamin A is given in terms of International Units (I.U.). Little of this vitamin is lost in normal cooking, but prolonged or repeated cooking will result in significant loss. The absorption of vitamin A and other fat-soluble vitamins requires bile acids, which are specific types of fat compounds stored in the gall bladder. Without these bile acids, all fat-soluble vitamins do not get properly absorbed into the blood, resulting in a vitamin deficiency. Table III shows which food sources contain vitamin A.

1. Vitamin A is effective in the treatment of chemically (methylcholanthrene) induced cancers in experimental animals and lung cancer in mice.[2,3] The growth of human breast cancer cells is decreased by vitamin A.[4] Vitamin A also inhibits the growth of human melanoma cells, a deadly skin cancer.[5] Several different clinical trials using vitamin A treatment for patients with skin, cervix, or lung cancer have been done in Europe and show very promising results.[6] Another study shows that vitamin A exerts a protective effect against lung cancers for smokers and nonsmokers.[7] Presently, there are clinical trials ongoing at the National Cancer Institute in Bethesda, Maryland, and other centers involving retinoic acid (vitamin A derivative) and its effect on patients with many types of cancer.

2. It maintains the integrity of the skin and all inner linings of the airways and gastrointestinal tract, the first line of defense against invading bacteria and other microorganisms.

3. Deficiency results in decreased production of antibodies to certain foreign substances like diphtheria and tetanus.[8] By giving enough vitamin A, antibody production is increased substantially. Impaired production of antibodies to cancer cells is also a possibility if vitamin A is at low levels in the blood.

4. Deficiency causes a decrease in T cells, which consequently renders the person at risk of not being able to kill cancer cells.

5. Deficiency enhances the binding of a certain carcinogen benzo(a)pyrene to respiratory cells' DNA in our lungs,[9] which in turn can transform the normal lung cell into a cancer cell.

6. Needed for proper color vision and night vision. Deficiency is the principal cause of blindness in the world.

7. Required for proper growth and maintenance of bones, teeth, glands, nails, and hair.

Vitamin A is one of the few vitamins that may lead to toxicity if taken in great excess. Typical symptoms include drowsiness, headache, vomiting, drying of the skin, and it may raise blood cholesterol and triglyceride levels. Daily doses of 100,000 I.U. (30 mg of retinol) have been given to adults for many months without serious side effects.[10] But children who ingest 50,000 to 500,000 I.U. (15 to 150 mg of retinol) per day do exhibit toxicity.[11] Based on this information, it seems reasonable for a healthy person to take up to 20,000 I.U. (6 mg of retinol) per day with relative safety.

Vitamin D

Vitamin D (cholecalciferol) requirements are now expressed in International Units (I.U.). Ten micrograms of cholecalciferol equal 400 I.U. of vitamin D. There are several types of vitamin D: some become activated when minimal ultraviolet light reacts with them in the skin; other types are activated by the liver or kidney. So if a person does not get minimal sunlight, or has liver or kidney disease, that person will be deficient in vitamin D (cholecalciferol). Most people get little or no vitamin D from their diet, but rather obtain their supply from production by skin cells after activation by ultraviolet light. Table III lists its food sources.

1. Vitamin D helps the body use calcium and phosphorus to build, form, and maintain all bones and teeth.

2. Vitamin D prevents rickets, a disease which distorts the growth of bones. (Cod liver oil was used as a folk remedy in Scotland in the eighteenth century and ultimately was found to have beneficial effects in the treatment of rickets.)

3. It has no known direct anticancer effect or direct action on the immune system other than to maintain the proper blood level of calcium, which is absolutely needed for the proper function of all killing cells in the body.

Toxicity may occur with large amounts of vitamin D. Fat-soluble vitamins, in contrast to water-soluble vitamins, are not rapidly broken down and disposed of quickly by the body. The earliest toxic symptoms are loss of appetite in children, nausea and vomiting, thirst, and constipation alternating with diarrhea. However, a daily dose of 100,000 to 150,000 I.U. of vitamin D (250 to 375 micrograms of cholecalciferol) for many months can be tolerated by a healthy adult.[14] Even so, there is no need to exceed the RDA of 400 I.U. of vitamin D (10 micrograms).

Vitamin E

Vitamin E requirements are now given as International Units where 1 I.U. equals 1 mg of dl-tocopherol. As we discussed in the chapter on free radicals, vitamin E is very important to us because it is an antioxidant. There is no difference between natural vitamin E and "d" vitamin E. The "d" denotes the chemical structure of the vitamin E molecule. Two preparations which contain identical amounts of natural vitamin E and dl-tocopherol are identical in their tocopherol content. (The natural preparation is usually more expensive.)

I would like to clear up a few myths about vitamin E. Vitamin E has been touted as the great "sex vitamin." There is no absolute proof about this except that rats which are deficient in vitamin E fail to reproduce. Vitamin E has not been shown to make a man more potent or to increase a woman's sex drive. As you know, sexual performance is a complex interaction between psychological and physical factors. In addition, vitamin E probably does not slow down the aging process per se; there is certainly no strong evidence for this. But it is a potent antioxidant, and aging is thought to be a process of oxidation (oxygen reacting with body tissues). Thirdly, there is some evidence that the elderly can walk longer distances after six months of supplemental vitamin E, but good studies concerning this have not yet been done.

Vitamin E has many important functions:

1. It is a potent antioxidant and as such acts as a scavenger, damaging free radicals which may produce cancer. Many studies have been done concerning the effect of vitamin E on the inhibition of cancer.[13,14,15] The results show that vitamin E can inhibit the growth of certain cancer cells.
2. As an antioxidant, it may directly protect a person against the cancer-inducing effects of smog. This protective effect has already been shown for animals.
3. It protects the body against the oxidation of polyunsaturated fatty acids. Therefore, it is essential that a person take enough vitamin E if his diet contains polyunsaturated fats. As you recall, polyunsaturated fats help to reduce the amount of blood cholesterol.
4. Vitamin E is essential for the normal function of red blood cells. A deficiency causes an anemia in children.
5. Vitamin E is beneficial for a very common breast disease, fibrocystic breast disease, which affects 50 percent of all women. This is a benign condition in which cysts develop, usually in both breasts, giving the breasts a granular consistency, and often associated with pain. However, women with fibrocystic disease have a two- to eightfold greater risk of developing breast cancer.[16,17] Several recent studies report that 85 percent

of women (twenty-six in the study group) with fibrocystic disease who took 600 I.U. of vitamin E daily for eight weeks experienced relief of the pain associated with their disease, and some of these women had demonstrable regression of disease.[18,19] The women whose disease did not respond had lower vitamin E levels when checked, suggesting a defect in vitamin E absorption.

6. Vitamin E reduces the LDL level (lipids involved in atherosclerosis) and increases the HDL level (lipids which protect against atherosclerosis). However, before everyone rushes to start taking vitamin E for its potential protective effect against heart disease, large population studies must be done to see if vitamin E consistently affects LDL and HDL in the same manner as it did in the small study cited (the findings were part of the fibrocystic breast disease study mentioned above).

There is no case on record of vitamin E toxicity nor any indication of vitamin E toxicity. A daily intake of 800 I.U. of vitamin E per 2.2 pounds of body weight for five months has not been toxic. This amounts to 56,000 I.U. (56,000 mg) for an average man weighing 140 pounds, or about 5600 times the RDA. A good dose of daily vitamin E seems to be 400 to 600 I.U. (400 to 600 mg).

Vitamin K

Vitamin K is essential for normal blood clotting. After vitamin K gets into the blood via the bile fats, it helps manufacture clotting proteins in a normal liver. Bacteria that normally inhabit our intestine also make vitamin K, and we get much of our needed vitamin K from their production. If the liver is not working properly (as in alcoholism), clotting factors are not made, and the person is at risk of bleeding to death in certain circumstances. Anticoagulant drugs (Coumadin) are purposely given to interfere with the action of vitamin K in those patients who are generating blood clots which may lodge in their lungs and cause death.

WATER-SOLUBLE VITAMINS

Thiamine (B_1)

Thiamine deficiency causes beriberi, a disease which was more prevalent when the rice-milling industry spread across Asia. Thiamine is easily destroyed by heating, and grain and cereal foods may lose quite a bit of thiamine when they are milled. In the United States, thiamine deficiency syndromes occur almost exclusively in alcoholics because of a poor diet, or for that matter, in any person who does not consume a good diet.

Thiamine food sources are listed in Table III.

1. Immunologically, animals show an increased risk of infection with certain bacteria if they are deprived of thiamine.[20]
2. It helps the body to fully utilize carbohydrates by interaction with enzymes.
3. Thiamine deficiency causes loss of appetite, mental depression, "pins and needles" sensation in the feet and hands and other sensory losses, and if very deficient, will cause beriberi.
4. It is required for the proper function of the heart.

There are no recorded cases of thiamine toxicity. Supplemental thiamine is recommended for all persons who are eating a poor diet.

Riboflavin (B_2)

Riboflavin is important because it is involved in so many chemical processes and functions in the body. Riboflavin in food must first be converted into an active form in the body before it can be used. Several drugs and diseases interfere with this conversion and hence will cause its deficiency.

1. Riboflavin deficiency results in a decrease in lymphocytes and an increased susceptibility to certain infections.[21] With T cells decreased, a person could also be more susceptible to cancer development.

2. It is essential for building and maintaining body tissues including the brain, blood, and skin.

3. It helps to transform proteins, fats, and carbohydrates into energy.

4. Riboflavin protects the body from skin disorders, cataracts and other corneal disorders.

5. Its deficiency can result from a low-protein diet and can cause lip, mouth, and tongue soreness and burning.

6. Excess thyroid hormone can use up riboflavin more quickly.

7. Boric acid, which is a part of some mouthwashes, suppositories, and some important foods, causes riboflavin to be secreted into the urine and thereby causes partial riboflavin deficiency.

Niacin

A diet deficient in niacin produces pellagra in humans. At one time, pellagra was endemic in Europe and America because the main diet consisted of cornmeal, molasses, and pork fat almost exclusively.

1. Niacin converts food to energy.

2. It prevents pellagra, a disease which affects the central nervous system, skin, and gastrointestinal tract.

3. Niacin has been given to patients to lower blood lipids, but it is not very effective for this.

4. There are no good studies to show that it stimulates the flow of blood around the body, especially the brain, for which niacin is frequently advocated.

Pantothenic Acid

Rarely is a human diet ever deficient in this important vitamin, because pantothenic acid is distributed in almost all plant and animal tissues. It has the following functions:

1. It is required in almost all energy-producing reactions in the body involving fats, carbohydrates, and proteins.

2. It is required for the formation of some hormones and nerve-regulating substances.

3. It helps to regulate the blood sugar level.

Pyridoxine (B_6)

Like most other B-complex vitamins, pyridoxine is not stored in the human body to any great extent. But even so, a deficiency in this vitamin is extremely rare. It has the following uses.

1. Pyridoxine has a marked effect on the immune system. Its deficiency inhibits the formation of antibodies, decreases the number of T cells, and decreases the ability of the immune system to reject foreign tissues like transplants[22] and to destroy cancer cells.

2. It is important in the formation of certain proteins and in the use of fats in the body.

3. Pyridoxine is essential for the proper function of the nervous system.

4. It is needed for the formation of red blood cells and for healthy gums and teeth.

5. More than the normal amount of pyridoxine is required by women who are using an oral contraceptive containing estrogen.

Vitamin B_{12}

Vitamin B_{12} has been known for over fifty years.

1. It is needed to make hemoglobin and other parts of the red blood cell.

2. B_{12} is required for healthy nervous tissue and normal growth.

3. A deficiency causes anemia and mental changes.

4. Many alcoholics develop vitamin B_{12} deficiency.

Folic Acid

1. Folic acid is essential for forming certain proteins and genetic materials in the body.

2. Its deficiency results in an anemia.

3. It is very important during the last three months of pregnancy.

Biotin

Biotin has only recently been discovered.

1. It synthesizes fatty acids, metabolizes carbohydrates for energy use, and makes the body use protein properly.

2. It aids in maintaining muscles, the circulatory system, nervous system, hair and skin, reproductive system, adrenal glands, and the thyroid gland.

3. Its deficiency results in depression, anemia, sleepiness, and muscle pain.

Vitamin C

Vitamin C is a major factor in controlling and potentiating multiple aspects of human resistance to many agents including cancer. Much work concerning vitamin C and its effects on infections and cancer has been done by Dr. Linus Pauling. However, some of the studies concerning vitamin C and cancer are controversial. Vitamin C is an antioxidant, and as such has tremendous implications in the management of free radicals, which can lead to the development of cancer. Curiously, the human is one of the few animals that does not manufacture its own vitamin C.

What is known about vitamin C is the following:

1. Vitamin C prevents the formation of nitrosamines (a potent carcinogen) from nitrites and amines, both in the test tube and in the body.[23,24]

2. Several studies show that vitamin C in foods, like lettuce,

is responsible for the decreased incidence of human gastric cancer in the U.S.[25]

3. Numerous studies show that vitamin C protects the body against human bladder cancer[26,27] and destroys another very potent bladder carcinogen called N-methyl-N-nitroso-guanidine.[28] People who take high doses of vitamin C excrete most of it in the urine, where nitrosamines are also excreted. This high amount of vitamin C which accumulates in the bladder neutralizes nitrosamines which would otherwise cause bladder cancer.

4. Vitamin C protects the body against most carcinogenic hydrocarbons.

5. Vitamin C is needed to produce collagen, a substance which gives structure to the bones, cartilage, muscles, and vascular tissues.

6. It may be needed in large amounts to protect the body from cancer by walling the cancer off from the rest of the body. This special wall is formed by collagen.[29]

7. Vitamin C molecules may inhibit cancer from spreading by neutralizing an enzyme (hyaluronidase) made by cancer cells which would otherwise help the cancer to metastasize.[30] It has been found that many cancer patients have low blood levels of vitamin C, but it is not known whether this is a result of poor nutrition, which is generally seen in cancer victims, or whether this is due to the fact that vitamin C is being used up to neutralize that special enzyme made by the cancer.

8. Smoking decreases the amount of vitamin C in lung tissue and blood. Here again, vitamin C could be neutralizing the toxic carcinogens contained in cigarette smoke.

9. Some animal studies by Homer Black show that vitamin C can reverse the carcinogenic effect of ultraviolet light.

10. The literature is replete with studies showing that vitamin C may have a protective role in viral illnesses. This information takes on new dimensions because we know that some

viruses can cause cancer in animals, and hence vitamin C may inhibit these cancers. Some human cancers are strongly suspected of being caused by viruses, but it is not absolutely proven. In these cases, vitamin C may have a protective role as well, but this is merely speculation at this time.

11. Vitamin C greatly affects the immune system: (a) the phagocytes require vitamin C for proper function; (b) a deficiency in vitamin C causes a decrease in T cells, the killing cells of the immune system.

The question is, how much vitamin C should a person take? It seems that large doses of vitamin C (large relative to that amount recommended by the RDA) can be taken without serious side effects. One way to estimate the amount of vitamin C we need is to measure the amount made by an animal which can manufacture it, and then extrapolate from that figure the amount a human needs based on body weight.[31] If an animal that makes X amount of vitamin C weighs 15 pounds and a human weighs 150 pounds, then the human's need of vitamin C is ten times X. Using this comparison, the estimate for a human's need for vitamin C is 2 to 4 grams without stress and up to 10 grams with stress. These amounts are many times higher than the RDA allowance of 60 milligrams. Dr. Pauling is reported to take about 10 grams of vitamin C daily. A study by Hoffer shows that doses of 3 to 30 grams of vitamin C in more than 1000 patients since 1953 did not cause one miscarriage, kidney stone formation, or any other serious toxicity.[32] Klenner has given patients 10 grams of vitamin C daily for over thirty years without any serious toxic side effects.[33]

DRUGS AND VITAMINS

The interaction between many drugs and nutrients has become known during the past fifteen years. Some of these drug

Table IV

EFFECT OF DRUGS ON NUTRITION*

Drug	Use	Vitamin Decreased
Anticonvulsants	Prevents seizures	Folic acid Vitamin D Vitamin K
Colchicine	Treats gout	Vitamin B_{12}
Coumadin	"Thins" blood	Vitamin K
Estrogen-containing oral contraceptives	Prevents conception	Folic acid Vitamin B_6, B_{12} Riboflavin Thiamine Vitamin C
Hydralazine	Treats hypertension	Vitamin B_6
Irritant laxatives	Laxative	Vitamin D
Isoniazid	Treats tuberculosis	Vitamin B_6 Niacin
Mineral oil	Laxative	Vitamin A Vitamin K Vitamin D
Para-aminosalicylic acid	Treats tuberculosis	Vitamin B_{12}
Tetracycline	Antibiotic	Vitamin C
Triamterene	Diuretic	Folic acid
Trimethoprim	Antibiotic	Folic acid

* From Ovesen, L. 1979. *Drugs* 18:278.

interactions involve the absorption or utilization of vitamins by the body and ultimately compromise a patient's health. Table IV provides a list of some commonly used prescription drugs, what they are used for, and the vitamins that the drugs interfere with. A patient who is taking one of these drugs should be aware that his or her diet may have to be supplemented with the indicated vitamin. Of course, if one of these drugs is taken for just a short period of time (like tetracycline) no vitamin supplementation is needed. However, if some drugs are taken for months or years (like anticonvulsants, birth control pills, high blood pressure pills, or antituberculosis drugs), then vitamin supplementation should be instituted.

MINERALS

Selenium

Selenium, a metal in our body, has three very important functions. First, selenium together with glutathione peroxidase is a major antioxidant and as such is a free radical scavenger; and it also enables organisms to survive with less oxygen. Second, selenium reacts with toxic metals to form biologically inert compounds. The metals that are toxic to our bodies but are rendered harmless by selenium are mercury, cadmium, and arsenic. Third, there is a correlation between night vision and the selenium content of the retina; the higher the selenium content, the better the vision.

Selenium could be obtained by a diet rich in whole-grain cereals, organ meats (liver, etc.), and seafoods. However, whole-grain cereals vary greatly in selenium content. It has been shown by G. N. Schrauzer and colleagues that the selenium content in pasteurized milk in Caracas, Venezuela, is ten times greater than in milk in Beltsville, Maryland.[34] Schrauzer and colleagues also studied the number of cancer deaths related to the amount of dietary selenium intake from food consumption in twenty-seven different countries and nineteen different states in the U.S.[35] They have concluded that the higher the blood selenium content, the lower the cancer incidence. The cancer incidence for each state, which is given in Chapter 1, correlates well with their selenium data. R. J. Shamberger has shown that selenium suppresses the development of skin tumors in animals.[36] Shamberger and Willis have shown that in 1965, the higher the soil or crop level of selenium, the lower the cancer death rate was in the United States and Canada.[37] They also studied the population in several American cities and found that the higher the average blood selenium level, the lower the cancer death rate.[38]

Another study demonstrates that rats which were depleted of selenium and fed a diet high in polyunsaturated fats developed breast cancer.[39] My own research shows that selenium protects the cell membrane from attack by free radicals. Other research by R. Medina and colleagues shows that selenium fed daily to mice inhibits cancer from forming in them.[40] The antioxidant property of selenium protects the body against cancer especially if the diet is high in polyunsaturated fats.

Several studies indicate that selenium deficiency corresponds to heart attacks.[41,42] High rates of heart disease and heart attacks are evident in selenium-deprived children in China and in selenium-deprived adults in Finland. Deaths from heart attack are highest in Finland, New Zealand, and perhaps South Africa. These countries have widespread selenium deficiency compared to the United States. When selenium supplements are given to Chinese children, significant improvement occurs in their heart disease rates.

Survival rates of offspring in animals is very sensitive to the amount of selenium in the mother. An average sow has four or five piglets per litter in areas of Finland with low selenium soil content. But when 0.1 mg of selenium is added to the diet, the litter size increases to ten.

Schrauzer maintains that the average selenium intake of the

American population is only one half of the amount required "for optimal protection against neoplastic [cancer] disease.[43] The average U.S diet contains between 50 and 160 micrograms of selenium per day, depending on where one lives. The recent recommendation by the National Research Council for selenium consumption is between 50 and 200 micrograms per day, but Schrauzer concludes from his studies that at least 300 micrograms of selenium per day is needed for cancer protection. Selenium toxicity occurs after prolonged ingestion of 2400 to 3000 micrograms of selenium per day.[44]

Obviously, selenium is not the only factor involved in cancer development or its progression, and it would be unwarranted to consume a great deal of selenium every day thinking that it alone would prevent cancer. However, depending upon where you live, a person could take supplemental selenium in the amount of 100 to 200 micrograms per day, assuming that you are living in an area which is adequate in selenium content and assuming that you are eating a well-balanced diet. Vegetarians, dieters, and people living in areas of the country without adequate selenium stores will require about 200 micrograms of selenium per day. A study shows that a total of 500 micrograms of selenium per day is safely tolerated by people in Japan.[45] Organic selenium, as found in certain yeasts, is better than inorganic selenium for supplementation because it has less systemic toxicity at high concentrations, it resists chemical changes, and it is stable during food processing.

Zinc

Zinc is a metal which is essential for good growth and development, protein synthesis, wound healing, and is a functional part of many enzymes. Danbolt and Closs have shown that zinc deficiency directly produces the symptoms and problems of an inherited disease called acrodermatitis enteropathica, which consists of multiple skin and gastrointestinal problems.[46] This disease is completely cured by dietary zinc supplementation.

More importantly, zinc is intimately involved in the immune system's function and cancer. This subject has been extensively reviewed by Robert A. Good and colleagues.[47] Zinc has the following effects:

1. Zinc deficiency decreases the number of T cells and suppressor T cells,[48,49] which could potentially lead to the development of cancer.
2. However, phagocytes are more efficient with low blood levels of zinc.[50]
3. Zinc deficiency is seen in patients with several different types of cancers, but this is related to poor dietary habits rather than to the cancer itself.
4. Zinc excess and zinc deficiency have both been shown to inhibit tumor growth in animals. Whereas zinc deficiency stimulates anticancer inflammatory cells, zinc-supplemented animals have augmented T cell anticancer activity.

Other Minerals

There are many other minerals required by our body to function properly. These include iodine, calcium, copper (an antioxidant), phosphorus, fluoride, manganese, magnesium, chromium, molybdenum, and others. All have important roles to ensure that all aspects of the body run smoothly. A chronic deficiency of iodine can cause thyroid cancer (one can use iodine-supplemented salt as a safeguard). Calcium is needed in many chemical reactions and is absolutely required for the proper functioning of the immune system, which includes killing T cells and complement proteins. Iron is needed for the synthesis of hemoglobin, the complex structure inside the red blood cell which transports oxygen throughout the body.

LOWERING THE RISK

Cancer patients have vitamin deficiencies (in particular folic acid, vitamin C, and pyridoxine) as well as other nutritional deficiencies.[51] There have been a number of studies of patients with proven cancer who are being treated with vitamin therapy alone. Many of these vitamin therapy studies have recently been reviewed by Bertino,[52] who concludes that such treatment is without proven benefit to the cancer patient—and this author agrees with him. The cancer patient should be thoroughly worked up by an oncology specialist, preferably at a good medical center. I am advocating simple common sense: an apparently healthy person should take steps to avoid or eliminate risk factors which could potentially cause cancer and atherosclerosis. This includes eating the right foods and taking the right amount of those vitamins and minerals shown to have anticancer and antioxidant effects, and shown to be needed for the immune system to function well. By eliminating all known risk factors of cancer and atherosclerosis and practicing good nutrition supplemented with vitamins and minerals, your overall risk of developing cancer or atherosclerosis will be kept to a minimum.

Richard S. Schweiker, Secretary of Health and Human Services, said in a policy statement given at a symposium on cancer research at Rockefeller University that he and the Reagan Administration endorse the research focus on cancer prophylaxis and the protective potential of vitamins and trace minerals in both normal and high-risk populations. As reported by the *Medical Tribune* on June 30, 1982, he said that enough new data have emerged in recent basic, clinical, and epidemiologic studies to justify support for the hypothesis that micronutrients may prevent the initiation or development of cancer. The National Cancer Institute in Bethesda, Maryland, has allocated several million dollars for this purpose.

Secretary Schweiker said, "This new strategy holds promise for reducing the incidence of cancer more successfully than an attempt to remove from the environment all substances which may initiate the cancer process—an approach which is not always possible or practical." In addition he said that laboratory studies of vitamin A precursors, vitamins C and E, selenium, and certain chemicals demonstrate that these "act as preventive agents."

I recommend the following combination of vitamins and minerals as a food supplement for the reasons outlined in this chapter. I call it the "Risk Modifier™." It could be taken daily unless otherwise specified by your physician. Children under 12 and pregnant or lactating women should not take it unless approved by their physician. The Risk Modifier™ for children is shown.

RISK MODIFIER

	Risk Modifier™		Risk Modifier™, Ages 1–4	
Vitamin or Mineral	**Dosage**	**% U.S. RDA**	**Dosage**	**% U.S. RDA**
Beta-carotene	16,666 I.U.† (10 mg)	333	—	—
Vitamin A (palmitate)	5,000 I.U.	100	2,500 I.U.	100
Vitamin D (cholecalciferol)	400 I.U.	100	400 I.U.	100
Vitamin E (dl-tocopherol)	500 I.U.	1665	20 I.U.	200
Vitamin C (ascorbic acid)	650 mg	1083	60 mg	150
Folic acid	400 mcg	100	.2 mg	100
Thiamine (B_1)	10 mg	670	1.1 mg	157
Riboflavin (B_2)	10 mg	588	1.28 mg	160
Niacin	20 mg	100	9.0 mg	100
Pyridoxine (B_6)	10 mg	500	1.12 mg	160
Cyancobalamin (B_{12})	18 mcg	300	4.50 mcg	150
Pantothenic acid	10 mg	100	5.0 mg	100
Biotin	300 mcg	100	151.0 mcg	100
Selenium (organic, yeasts)	200 mcg	*	50.0 mcg	*
Copper (cupric oxide)	3 mg	150	1.25 mg	125
Zinc	24 mg	160	10.0 mg	125

RISK MODIFIER—*Continued*

	Risk Modifier™		Risk Modifier™, Ages 1–4	
Vitamin or Mineral	**Dosage**	**% U.S. RDA**	**Dosage**	**% U.S. RDA**
Iodine	150 mcg	100	70.0 mcg	100
Calcium	—	—	15 mg	1.8
Phosphorus	—	—	7.5 mg	.9
Iron	—	—	6.0 mg	4.0
Magnesium	—	—	7.5 mg	5.0
Manganese gluconate	—	—	0.5 mg	40

* Established as adequate and safe by the National Research Council, National Academy of Sciences, but no RDA has been established yet.

† Can be converted to vitamin A according to body needs where 10 mg of beta-carotene is equivalent to 16.666 I.U. of vitamin A.

THREE

The Risks

7

Food Additives and Contaminants

CHEMICAL food additives and food contaminants have been quite extensively studied, more so than most other chemicals that come into contact with our bodies—with good reason. Only carefully selected chemicals can prevent contamination and spoilage of food that has to be produced in great quantities, stored, and transported. Chemicals are also used for flavoring and appearance. Chemical contaminants may occur as a result of food processing procedures such as irradiation, cooking, pickling, or smoking. The trouble with the use of chemicals in food is that we are exposed to them constantly, repeatedly, and at low doses. For this reason it is difficult to ascertain from tests whether these chemicals can cause cancer, and therefore the decision whether or not they are potentially hazardous must be made from laboratory investigations rather than large population studies.

Chemical food additives are divided into several groups. *Intentional* food additives are chemicals which are purposely added to food. Some of these definitely produce cancers in animals, but others do not produce such clear results. Thiourea[1] and butter yellow[2] produce cancers in animals and are no longer used in food. A very important antioxidant presently used in foods, butylated hydroxytoluene, is reported to enhance certain animal cancers[3] but inhibit some carcinogens.[4] Red

No. 2 and Red No. 40 dyes have both been banned because they are not safe according to the Food and Drug Administration.

Cyclamate has not been shown to be carcinogenic in humans, but its metabolite does produce testicular atrophy (shrinking) in rats. Saccharin, another highly publicized intentional food additive, does produce bladder cancer in rats when given at 5 percent or more in the diet,[5] but epidemiological studies show that saccharin does not pose a major cancer risk to man.[6] However, it is generally agreed that additional studies are needed concerning the effects of saccharin on man before conclusive statements can be made. Xylitol, a new sweetener compound, also has been reported to give rise to bladder cancer in mice and adrenal cancer in rats.[7]

Nitrite is a most important food additive. Nitrites are used as meat preservatives to prevent botulism; they also add color to certain meats, especially bacon and hot dogs. Nitrites can react with other compounds to form potent carcinogens called nitrosamines.[8] When bacon is cooked, nitrosamines form. Look at the label of ingredients on your package of bacon or hot dogs—nitrites are probably listed. There is a low level of nitrites in our saliva and in some vegetables, but there is no information whether these nitrites can be activated to form nitrosamines. Vitamin C, also found in vegetables, can inhibit the formation of nitrosamines and is usually added to meat cures. Some research has suggested that nitrite itself might be carcinogenic.[9]

A certain wine additive, diethylpyrocarbonate, interacts with alcohol to cause levels of 0.1 parts per billion of another strong carcinogen, urethan.[10] This chemical is banned in many countries now.

Unintentional food additives are those chemicals used to prepare or store the food product; small amounts of these chemicals subsequently, unintentionally, become part of the food. An example of this is trichloroethylene. Decaffeinated products were made by using trichloroethylene to extract the caffeine. Trichloroethylene was found to be a carcinogen and was removed from the market. Another example of unintentional contamination of food involves certain processes used to make the paraffin wax which lines many food containers. Carcinogens were formed during certain of these processes, and once discovered, these processes were discontinued. Pesticides like DDT, aldrin, and others produce liver cancer in mice but do not appear to be carcinogenic for other species (although they are highly toxic). However, it is important to realize that most pesticides get into our bodies and are stored in fat cells, since they are fat soluble. These pesticide-laden fat cells can then act as reservoirs to slowly, but constantly, release the pesticide into the blood stream. Another chemical which is used in agriculture is DES (diethylstilbestrol). DES is used for cattle and has been found in trace amounts in foods derived from cattle. DES causes human cancer: cancer of the vagina in young women and cancer of the testicles in men, whose mothers had taken DES. (Cancer of the testicles is rare, however, especially in this situation.) It must be kept in mind that there is a very great difference in the amount of DES needed to cause cancer (which is very large) and that amount that contaminates our food (which is very little).

Some food contaminants, like aflatoxin, which causes human liver cancer, are of natural origin. It is a product of a fungus, *Aspergillus flavus,* which grows mainly on peanut plants. Other fungal products have been implicated in human cancers, but have not yet been substantiated. *Gyromita esculenta,* a common mushroom used in cooking, contains a compound called N-methyl-N-formylhydrazine, which is a most potent animal carcinogen.[11] Related chemicals in other mushroom types are now under investigation. There is no current information on cancer incidence related to the amount of mushrooms eaten by people in different parts of the world.

FOOD PROCESSING

Certain food processing techniques, such as smoking and charcoal broiling, are known to produce carcinogens.[12] Smoked food is associated with an increased incidence of gastric cancer in the Baltic states and Iceland. The carcinogens which result from charcoal broiling appear to come from fat which drips from the meat and is burned, forming the carcinogen, which then rises with the smoke back up into the meat.[13] If the fat drippings were eliminated, the carcinogens would probably be eliminated also.

As yet there are no definite proven cases of human cancers directly related to food additives, but many authorities agree that additives and contaminants do account for a very small percentage of human cancers. Those chemicals implicated in causing animal cancers were removed from the market for the most part. However, nitrites are bothersome sources of carcinogens and should be avoided. It is altogether possible that the reduced incidence of gastric cancer in the United States is directly related to better methods of food preparation and smaller amounts of nitrites being used in foods. Also it seems that certain naturally occurring food components like aflatoxins do cause human cancer and should definitely be eliminated. And finally, think twice before you make a habit of eating a great many mushrooms.

8

Obesity

OBESITY affects about 35 percent of all Americans. Being obese carries with it a social stigma as well as a general health risk. One study calculated that there are 832 million pounds of excess fat in American men and 1468 million pounds of excess fat in American women, for a total of 2.3 billion pounds.[1] That is a staggering amount of fat, and it has been increasing over the past several decades. More obesity occurs in middle-aged people and in people with low socioeconomic status. The percentage of black American women who are obese is greater than the percentage of white women. Obesity runs in families, and adopted children become obese if adoptive family members are obese—hence, probably both genetic and environmental factors influence the development of obesity.

The fat cell *size* is increased in all types of obesity. An increased *number* of fat cells is found in children and adults who were obese before the age of 2. Statistics show that if a child is obese before he is 2 years old, he will likely be obese in adulthood because he already has an increased number of fat cells. It is ideal, then, not to allow a baby to become fat, because if he does, the resulting fat cells will remain with him for the rest of his life. Adult obese patients who have an increased number of fat cells acquired before age 2 are usually more grossly obese and will have obesity in the abdomen and chest as well as in the forearm. It is more difficult for an obese patient to lose weight if he was obese before age 2; in other words, it is more difficult for an obese patient to lose weight if he has more fat cells than normal. Ninety-nine percent of all obesity is directly related to overeating—make no mistake about that! Only 1 percent of obesity is caused by a disease or a medical problem.

Because obese individuals tend to develop a variety of diseases, some of which are life-threatening, obese adults have a higher than normal death rate for their age group. The risk of death correlates almost directly with how much a person is overweight. Even if you are only a little overweight, you still have an increased risk of death compared to a person who is not overweight.

There have been several studies to suggest that longevity is correlated with factors that limit the adult body size. In 1935, C. M. McCay showed that feeding rats a low-protein diet yielded lean animals that lived much longer than animals fed high-protein diets.[2] Many more of these types of experiments were completed or are in progress by Dr. Robert A. Good and colleagues at Memorial Sloan-Kettering Hospital in New York City.[3,4] They have had similar results: animals with lean body mass live much longer. In addition, investigations by Tannenbaum,[5] Kraybill,[6] and others[7,8,9] have shown that animals with lean body masses have lower rates of cancer development as well as greater longevity. Because of all these well-planned studies, the National Dairy Council issued the following statement in 1975: "Of all dietary modification studies, caloric restriction has had the most regular influence on the genesis of neoplasms in experimental animals."[10]

Obesity is a major risk factor for the development of endometrial cancer (cancer of the inner lining of the uterus) in postmenopausal women. The reason for this is that obese postmenopausal women produce a lot more of a female hormone called estrone. This increased production is directly related to the number and size of the woman's fat cells, since estrone is manufactured in the fat cells from another hormone (androstenedione). Estrone constantly stimulates the uterus, and this is believed to cause endometrial cancer. Similarly, postmenopausal women who take estrogens daily for symptoms of menopause also have a higher incidence of endometrial cancer. The mechanism is presumably the same.

People who are obese usually consume more fats in their diet; this is a major risk factor for the development of breast cancer and colon cancer.[11] Both height and weight are positively associated with cancer in postmenopausal women. An animal study done recently showed that if food intake was reduced (the number of calories decreased) during a "critical period" after a carcinogen was given to induce breast cancer, then the development of the cancer was inhibited.[12] This may result from low amounts of two hormones, prolactin and estrogen. Leaner animals produce less of these two hormones, which in high amounts can lead to the development of cancer.

In addition, obesity can adversely affect the body's response to infection. Diets which are high in fat depress a person's resistance to tuberculosis, malaria, and pneumococcus (an often severe pneumonia). Obese animals have more severe infections and higher death rates from the infections.[13] The incidence of pneumonia is significantly higher in obese infants compared to nonobese infants.[14] Adverse effects on the immune system or poor lung ventilation due to obesity have been suggested as possible reasons for severe pneumonias in these infants.

An obese person also has a two or three times higher risk of developing diabetes. Obesity interferes with the action of insulin, the hormone that normally packs sugar into the cells of the body. Hence, with interference of insulin, the blood sugar level goes very high. If this person loses weight, insulin can then work properly and usually return the blood sugar level to normal.

An obese person has an increased risk of developing cardiovascular disease. The reasons for increased heart attacks are not clear but may be related to increased blood lipids associated with obesity. Obese people tend to have higher blood cholesterol and triglycerides. If the obese person loses weight, the high blood levels of cholesterol and triglyceride return to normal. Obese people have higher incidences of hypertension, which additionally contributes to the risk of heart attack and stroke.

Obesity contributes to the development of gall bladder disease and also is a risk factor for major respiratory problems. Some massively obese individuals have trouble breathing because the weight of the chest is so great that the individual's chest muscles have difficulty lifting it. Being overweight causes too much wear and tear on bone joints and leads to the early development of joint problems.

How much should a person weigh? There is no one answer, but here is a good rule of thumb. Men who are 5 feet tall should weigh 110 pounds. For every 1 inch over 5 feet, add another 5 pounds. Thus if a man is 5 feet 11 inches tall, his ideal weight is about 165 pounds. Women who are 5 feet tall should weigh about 100 pounds. For every 1 inch over 5 feet, add 5 pounds. Therefore, if a woman is 5 feet 6 inches tall, her ideal weight is about 130 pounds.

If you do need to lose weight, you should do it gradually. Losing one or two pounds a week is safe, and that loss will probably be maintained. Do not lose more weight than called for by the formula. Successful weight loss and maintenance of that loss will be achieved only if you totally modify your eating habits. Many people are put on high-protein liquid diets consisting of 800 calories a day and lose a great deal of weight within the first few weeks. But on a long-term basis, these pounds come right back on because the person did not learn new eating habits. Diets containing less than 800 calories per day may be dangerous if the person is not closely monitored by a physician. To lose weight, you must eat less and increase your physical activity. Before you start a physical exercise program, you should be checked by a physician. An exercise program should start out gradually, with new goals set every week. Walking is very good exercise. Every pound of fat you have contains about 3500 calories. Therefore, to lose one pound, you have to burn off 3500 calories more than you eat. You will lose a pound a week if you burn off 500 calories per day more than you consume. If you eat a diet containing 1200 calories per day and burn off 1700 calories per day, you will lose one pound a week. Refer to Table I in Chapter 16 for the number of calories in the various foods listed.

Table I below shows approximately how many calories are

Table I

Activity	Calories/hr Used
Sleeping	80
Sitting	100
Driving a car	120
Standing	140
Housework	180
Walking $2\frac{1}{2}$ mph	210
Bicycling $5\frac{1}{2}$ mph	210
Gardening	220
Golf, mowing lawn	250
Bowling	270
Walking $3\frac{3}{4}$ mph	300
Swimming $\frac{1}{4}$ mph	300
Volleyball	350
Chopping wood	400
Tennis	420
Skiing 10 mph	600
Handball and squash	600
Bicycling 13 mph	660
Running 10 mph	900

used up by a 150-pound person performing the indicated activity. This information comes from the Department of Agriculture in a 1980 publication derived from data prepared by Dr. Robert Johnson at the University of Illinois.

If you lose weight suddenly or without a good reason, see a physician. Unexplained weight loss could be a sign of cancer or other serious medical problem.

Even though it is very difficult to lose weight, you must try because of the tremendous benefits of being at your ideal weight. There are no benefits in being obese, and the risks are very great.

9

Smoking—Slow-Moving Suicide

SMOKING is one of the biggest health hazards today. The scientific evidence is tremendous. In 1979 Joseph Califano, then Secretary of the Department of Health, Education, and Welfare, wrote: "Smoking is the largest preventable cause of death in America." In 1979, over 55 million American men and women smoked 615 billion cigarettes; and worldwide consumption is about 3 trillion each year. Since then regular cigarette smoking by adults has dropped slightly from 40 percent to about 33 percent. Whereas the percentage of adult male smokers decreased from 50 to 38 percent between 1964 and 1978, the percentage of adult female smokers remained the same at 30 percent. In the past two years, the percentages of both groups inched upward. The death rate from lung cancer for women in 1978 was three times higher than it was in 1964. Women today are more apt to smoke as much and in the same manner as men; these women have the same death rate and complications from lung cancer as men.

Smoking among children has increased dramatically. Since 1968, the number of girls between the ages of 12 and 14 who smoke has increased eightfold. Six million children between the ages of 13 and 19 are regular smokers, and over 100,000 children under 13 are now regular smokers. Smoking among blacks exceeds that of whites. However, on a positive note, about 30 million Americans have become ex-smokers since massive educational warnings were issued by the federal government.

More deaths and physical suffering are related to cigarette smoking than to any other single cause: over 125,000 deaths (and rising) each year from cancer, over 225,000 deaths from cardiovascular disease, and more than 20,000 deaths from chronic lung diseases. The cigarette industry's own research over a ten-year period (1964–1974), which cost over $15 million, confirmed the fatal dangers of smoking cigarettes.[1] In a one-year period, a one-pack-a-day smoker inhales 50,000 to 70,000 puffs which contain over 2,000 chemical compounds, many of which are known carcinogens. The president of the American Cancer Society, Dr. Robert V. P. Hutter, points out that many tobacco product ingredients, such as flavoring additives, are kept secret even from the government.

The cost of smoking-related diseases is staggering. Health care in the United States costs over $205 billion each year. The federal government pays about $60 billion of that. Smoking accounts for approximately $27 billion per year. A great deal of this cost is paid by nonsmokers and smokers through ever-increasing health insurance premiums, disability payments, and other programs. It doesn't seem fair that nonsmokers have to pay one penny for self-induced smokers' diseases.

The longer a person smokes, the greater is his risk of dying. A person who smokes two packs a day has a death rate two times higher than a nonsmoker. The earlier a person starts smoking, the higher is his risk of death compared to a smoker who begins later in life. Smokers who inhale have higher mortality rates than smokers who do not.

If a smoker stops smoking, his mortality rate decreases progressively as the number of nonsmoking years increase. Those who have stopped for fifteen years have similar mortality rates as those who never smoked, with the exception of smokers who stopped after the age of 65. Persons who smoke cigars and pipes also have an increased risk of death. Life expectancy is eight to nine years shorter for a two-pack-a-day smoker of age 30 to 35 compared to a nonsmoker, and those who smoke cigarettes with higher contents of "tar" and nicotine have a much higher death rate. Overall, the greatest mortality is seen in the 45 to 55 age groups. Hence, death from smoking is premature death!

SMOKING AND CANCER

Lung Cancer

Cigarette smoking is the major risk factor for lung cancer in both men and women. The scientific evidence for this and for other cancers related to smoking is overwhelming. The risk of developing lung cancer is increased by the amount of smoking, duration of smoking, age at which smoking started, and content of tar and nicotine. Female lung cancer deaths are rising at an alarming rate, and if this trend continues, it will become the leading cause of female cancer deaths. Smoking now accounts for 25 percent of all cancer deaths in women. The use of cigarettes with low tar and nicotine and the use of filters tend to decrease the number of lung cancer deaths when compared to smokers who use neither.

Evidence suggests that certain lung cancer cells come from precursor abnormal cells found in smokers.[2] These precursor cells are present for years before an overt cancer develops. A smoker who has only these precursor cells and no cancer cells can eliminate these precursor cells if he or she stops smoking. However, there is an undetermined point of no return at which time the precursor cell develops into a cancer cell—even if the person stopped smoking one day before this change occurs. After a single cancer cell develops, it may be many years before the cancer is detected.

Smoking acts in combination with certain occupational exposures to produce lung diseases. This combining effect is more than additive. However, in most of the studies done before 1964, adequate smoking histories were not obtained from the subjects, so many of the workers in mining industries (coal, hematite, copper) and refining (nickel, chromium) claimed that the industrial exposure itself produced the many lung diseases, from chronic bronchitis to cancer, for which they claimed compensation. It is probable that smoking had a great deal to do with the development of these "industrial diseases." There are several ways tobacco can act in combination with environmental factors to produce toxic chemicals and carcinogens. The tobacco plant itself can become contaminated with toxic chemicals such as insecticides. Some environmental toxicities, like coal, may increase a smoker's risk for developing disease. Synergism may occur: smoking and asbestos exposure may act together to greatly increase a person's risk of developing lung cancer. Also, those who smoke the most in general have the highest occupational incidence of other chemical exposure; that is, blue-collar workers smoke much more than white-collar workers.

There has been much concern about marijuana and its effects on the human body. The National Academy of Sciences released a report in 1982 entitled "Marijuana and Health," which states that there is a "strong possibility" that heavy marijuana smoking may lead to lung cancer. In fact, marijuana tar extracts have produced genetic changes in cells, and the smoke has 50 percent more carcinogenic hydrocarbons than cigarette smoke.

Nutrition and Lung Cancer

A study done by T. Hirayama showed that for those who smoked and also ate green and yellow vegetables every day, there was a slight beneficial effect when compared to a similar group of smokers who did not consume vegetables daily.[3] This is only one study and should not be taken to mean that a smoker is "safe" if he eats vegetables every day.

Other Tobacco-Related Cancers

Smoking cigarettes, pipes, and cigars is directly related to cancer of the larynx in men and women, and the more alcohol a smoker consumes, the higher is his risk of developing larynx cancer. Asbestos exposure has this same synergistic effect. Other cancers related to smoking include cancer of the mouth, esophagus, and pancreas, and here again, alcohol acts to intensify the effects of tobacco smoking. Cancer of the kidney and the urinary bladder are also directly related to smoking. Chewing tobacco or snuff-dipping in nonsmokers causes a fourfold increase of oral cancers and a sixfold increase in those who were both tobacco smokers and heavy alcohol drinkers.[4] Furthermore, countries such as India, Ceylon, China, and the Central Republics of the Soviet Union have the highest rates of death from oral cancer because the people there combine snuff and/or chewing tobacco with other ingredients such as betel nut. A chemical in the betel nut (N'nitrosonornicotine) can initiate tumors in animals. Hence these findings should discourage the use of chewing tobacco or snuff as a substitute for smoking, because a person simply exchanges one type of cancer risk for another.

Carcinogens of Tobacco Smoke

There are over 2,000 chemical compounds generated by tobacco smoke. The gas phase contains carbon monoxide, carbon dioxide, ammonia, nitrosamines, nitrogen oxides, hydrogen cyanide, sulfurs, nitriles, ketones, alcohols, and acrolein.

The "tars" contain extremely carcinogenic hydrocarbons which include nitrosamines, benzo(a)pyrenes, anthracenes, acridines, quinolines, benzenes, naphthols, naphthalenes, cresols, and insecticides (DDT), as well as some radioactive compounds like potassium-40 and radium-226.

Do any of these compounds look familiar? Compare this list with the list of chemicals known to be risk factors for human cancer, described in Chapter 2.

SMOKING AND CARDIOVASCULAR DISEASE

Smoking is one of the three major independent risk factors for cardiovascular diseases and intensifies the effects of other cardiac risk factors. Recently, Dr. A. Pic of the Haut Leveque Cardiac Hospital in Pessac, France, reported that a majority of a group of men under 35 years old who smoked more than thirty cigarettes a day had heart attacks immediately after vigorous exercise.[5] He warns that young athletes who smoke may be at an increased risk for heart disease.

There is extensive evidence to show that smoking is associated with more severe and more extensive atherosclerosis of the aorta and coronary heart arteries than in nonsmokers. This is probably related to the hydrocarbon carcinogens in cigarette smoke that have the potential to initiate the atherosclerotic process (see Chapter 2). Two chemical compounds in tobacco smoke, nicotine and carbon monoxide, can aggravate heart disease, chest pain, and other vascular symptoms. Carbon monoxide can significantly raise the blood hemoglobin concentration to dangerously high levels in smokers. If smoking is stopped, painful symptoms lessen, especially from compromised arteries of the legs. In addition, women who smoke and use birth control pills have a tenfold increased risk of cardiac disease.

SMOKING AND OTHER SERIOUS DISEASES

Chronic lung diseases related to smoking are second to coronary heart disease as a cause of disability. Chronic bronchitis and emphysema are seen much more often in smokers, and death from these diseases is higher when compared to nonsmokers. Respiratory symptoms, like cough and sputum production and lung function abnormalities, are seen in smokers, adults as well as young adolescents. If smoking is stopped, lung function and symptoms can improve.

Persons who smoke are two times more likely to develop peptic ulcer disease and death from peptic ulcers than are nonsmokers. Also, once an ulcer develops, smoking retards the healing process.

EFFECTS OF SMOKING ON PREGNANCY, INFANTS, AND GENETICS

The birth weight of a baby born to a woman who smoked during the pregnancy is considerably lower than the birth weight of a child of a nonsmoker. The more the mother smokes, the more the infant's birth weight decreases. This weight deficiency is due to retardation of growth, probably from the harmful effects of carbon monoxide, which decreases the amount of oxygen delivered to the fetus. Smoking during pregnancy may affect subsequent child development, physical growth, and mental development up to the age of 11 at least.

The risk of spontaneous abortion and of the fetus dying at birth are higher if the mother smoked during pregnancy, probably because there was less oxygen delivered to the fetus. There are more premature births and more deaths of these premature infants—and a higher incidence of the "sudden infant death syndrome"—in babies delivered from mothers who smoked during pregnancy.

Heavy cigarette smokers have a higher frequency of genetic abnormalities[6] and have a high frequency of sperm abnormalities,[7] the latter probably due to the genetic damage caused by smoking. In addition, smoking has a pronounced effect on some drugs, food products, and laboratory blood tests.

SMOKING AND THE IMMUNE SYSTEM

Smoking affects a person's immune system in several ways. People may have allergies to tobacco and tobacco smoke products, because there are definite antibodies made to some of these products. In addition, people who have other allergies (pollen, mold, dust) are much more sensitive to smoke than those who do not have such allergies. Another dramatic effect on a person's defenses is that smoking kills the hairlike structures (microcilia) which line the airways of the lungs. These hairs normally beat upwardly in a synchronous fashion to remove any debris and bacteria that may try to invade the lungs. Chronic smokers usually have severe colds and sometimes may develop pneumonia because smoking killed the microcilia that ordinarily would have protected them. And though there are more phagocytes in the lung tissue of smokers, they do not function properly. T lymphocytes also do not function properly in the smoker.

EFFECTS OF SMOKING ON A NONSMOKER

A nonsmoker who is exposed to tobacco smoke has many adverse reactions and is unjustly and unnecessarily subjected to risk factors detrimental to his or her health. The smoke that comes from the lighted end of a cigarette contains more hazardous chemicals than does the smoke that is inhaled by the smoker. A number of studies now indicate that carcinogenic, respiratory, and cardiovascular effects result from nonsmokers' exposure to indoor tobacco smoke.[8] In fact, wives of heavy smokers were found to have a higher risk of developing lung cancer than wives of nonsmokers.[9] The more cigarettes the husband smokes per day, the higher the risk for the wife. In addition, a study from the Surgeon General's Report of 1981 indicates that radioactive polonium 210 is found in tobacco and tobacco smoke. This radioactive material increases the risk for developing lung cancer in the nonsmoker.

Nonsmokers who are chronically exposed to smoke have small airway malfunctions, which cause many different lung diseases.[10] Children of parents who smoke have more bronchitis and pneumonia during the first year of their life. A majority of nonsmokers have eye and nose irritation when exposed to smoke, and the carbon monoxide from smoke causes nonsmokers to have less tolerance to exercise, less endurance, and decreased attentiveness.

Not only does the nonsmoker experience many harmful health effects from tobacco smoke, but he or she has to pay higher health insurance premiums for diseases related to smoking (cancer, cardiovascular diseases, lung diseases, etc.). Moreover, nonsmokers subsidize the tobacco industry through their tax dollars.

STOP SMOKING

More than 95 percent of former smokers quit on their own, usually at the recommendation of their physician. People who follow this popular strategy outlined by the American Lung Association have had good results:

1. Set a future date when you will stop smoking, and sign a contract with yourself to that effect.
2. Make a list of:
   a. All the reasons you continue to smoke ("It's a crutch," "It feels good")
   b. All your bonds with smoking (coffee, alcohol, etc.)
   c. All your reasons for not quitting
   d. All the reasons you should quit smoking
   e. All the rewards for becoming a nonsmoker
   f. Every cigarette you smoke for the two weeks before your quit date
   g. All situations you think will be difficult without a cigarette
3. Find substitutes for cigarettes, like chewing gum, etc.
4. Save your butts for two weeks before quitting day. Put

them in a jar and then fill the jar up with water and keep it in a visible place. Every time you feel the urge to smoke, open the jar and take a whiff.

5. Be prepared for withdrawal symptoms—cough, constipation, tiredness, headache, sore throat, trouble sleeping. These last only a week at most.

6. Begin a daily exercise program (walking, etc.) and eat the proper foods.

7. Tell all the people you know that you are going to quit and tell your friends how they can help.

8. Use coping techniques to break your smoking pattern:
   a. "I have the strength to do it."
   b. Doodle, stretch, touch your toes.
   c. Put a rubber band on your wrist and snap it every time you have the urge.
   d. Take a deep breath and hold it for several seconds and then exhale. Repeat this several times until the urge disappears.
   e. Avoid smoking situations and places; avoid people who smoke.
   f. Move around, take a shower, go get a drink, etc.
   g. Remember: "A craving for a cigarette will go away whether or not I smoke."

9. Don't dwell on your desire for a cigarette. Simply decide you have smoked your last cigarette.

10. Don't have in mind when the discomfort should end. Change your routine to distract yourself.

11. Sign a final nonsmoker contract with yourself.

A common mistake a "quitter" makes is to think it is all right to have one or two cigarettes every once in a while. If you could have done that before, you would have.

Your local chapter of the American Lung Association has courses on how to stop smoking. These sessions are inexpensive and quite comprehensive. I encourage you to use them.

Federally sponsored programs support tobacco prices, benefiting allotment holders (a unique monopoly situation) and tobacco growers. In addition, other federally sponsored programs benefit the tobacco industry. The programs and their cost to the taxpayer—both smoker and nonsmoker—are the following: tobacco inspection and grading, $6.1 million; market news service, $10.5 million; research, $7.4 million; short-term credit, $69.2 million (1979). Total cost to the taxpayer: over $157 million in 1979.

On the other hand, federal funds are spent to discourage smoking, to research the health effects of smoking, and to provide a great portion of the cost of medical care for people who are suffering from and dying of smoking-related diseases. Patients with *self-induced* smoking-related diseases and families of these patients receive Social Security benefits.

The United States has adopted uncompromisingly restrictive measures concerning food additives, but only a verbal statement of caution is required on every package of cigarettes. The Delaney Clause legislation prohibits the sale of any product to the American people that has been shown to be carcinogenic for humans and animals, and thus applies to situations in which the human hazard may be minimal. Tobacco is a major risk factor for cancer, cardiovascular diseases, lung diseases, and other illnesses. If you smoke, you should stop. If you have not started, don't! Seek professional help if you must, but stop smoking.

10

Alcohol and Caffeine

THE PRICE OF ALCOHOL ABUSE

INDUSTRIAL losses in the United States due to alcohol cost about $45 billion every year. Many more billions of dollars are added to this figure when one considers that alcohol is involved in 50 percent of all traffic fatalities, 30 percent of small-aircraft accidents, and 66 percent of all violent crimes. Furthermore, the totals are higher still when one considers the losses due to diseases aggravated by alcohol abuse, and losses due to alcohol-induced poor decision-making in government, industry, education, law, the military, and medicine. About 68 percent of adult Americans abuse alcohol.

Excessive alcohol consumption is a risk factor for mouth cancer, pharynx cancer, larynx cancer, esophagus cancer, pancreas cancer, liver cancer, and head and neck cancer. Alcohol acts synergistically with tobacco smoking in the development of other gastrointestinal cancers and urinary bladder cancer. A greater frequency of these cancers occurs in men, blacks, people on the low end of the socioeconomic scale, and older people. Alcohol is directly responsible for causing cirrhosis of the liver, which is the seventh leading cause of death in the United States. Fifty percent of deaths in alcoholics are due to cardiovascular diseases and 20 percent due to accidents, suicides, and homicides.

Nutrition and Alcoholism

Alcoholics have more nutritional deficiencies than all other groups of people.[1] Alcohol is a source of calories, and alcoholics consume this rather than foods with much better nutrient value. Alcoholics will consume about 20 percent of their total calories as alcohol.

Many vitamin deficiencies are severe in alcoholics. The most important is thiamine deficiency (vitamin B_1). A severe brain disease called Wernicke-Korsakoff syndrome can be rapidly reversed in alcoholics by the administration of thiamine. Folic acid and vitamin B_{12} deficiencies are seen in alcoholics due to the lack of fresh fruits and vegetables in their diets. These deficiencies are responsible for anemias, among other things. Pyridoxine (B_6) deficiency is responsible for alcoholics' peripheral nerve problems. Vitamin C is normally stored and activated in the liver, but alcoholics have a deficiency of vitamin C because of their liver disease. Because of vitamin deficiencies alcoholics complain of visual problems and sometimes infertility, since their sperm production may be impaired. In addition to vitamin deficiencies alcoholics have several mineral deficiencies including calcium, zinc, and magnesium. Since alcohol can interfere with the absorption of iron from the gut, some alcoholics develop the Plummer-Vinson syndrome, which is characterized by a cluster of symptoms including difficulty swallowing; a red, smooth tongue; and iron deficiency anemia. People with this syndrome have a high rate of cancer of the mouth.

Alcohol, Cancer, and Other Diseases

Alcohol may exert its carcinogenic effects by direct topical action on the mouth, pharynx, and esophagus. One study shows that alcohol consumption by women increases the risk of developing breast cancer when compared to nondrinkers.[2] The study did not say how much alcohol the women drank or how long they drank. Other studies are needed to corroborate this association. Alcohol and tobacco account for 75 percent of all oral cancers in the United States. And a considerable amount of evidence shows that alcoholism, because of the nutritional deficiencies associated with it, significantly increases the risk of smoking-related cancers.

The rate of liver cancer in alcoholics who have cirrhosis is rising. In addition, there are many other complications of cirrhosis, including varicose veins in the esophagus, which can bleed; ascites (fluid in the abdomen); muscle wasting; and kidney failure. Alcohol induces an inflammation of the pancreas and other abnormalities of the pancreas, and the heart can become severely enlarged and nonfunctional with alcoholism.

Alcoholics are much more prone to infections as well. Pneumonia is a common cause of death. Infections of the brain and heart are common. Alcoholics seem to have a defect in their T lymphocyte cell function, which may be reversible because it is probably related to nutritional deficiencies.[3] As you recall, normal T cells help to defend against cancer development.

Premature testicle and ovary shrinkage are seen in alcoholics. Peptic ulcers are also common and are often quite large. Infants born of alcoholic mothers may have a variety of problems including defects in the brain, in intellectual development and physical growth, and in the facial features. This is called the "fetal alcohol syndrome," in which alcohol acts to transform normal cells of the fetus into abnormal cells. The number of persons affected in this way is grossly underestimated.

CAFFEINE AND CANCER

Caffeine is the most popular drug in North America and in many other parts of the world. It is found in coffee, tea, cola beverages, and chocolate.

Coffee drinking may be related to cancer of the lower urinary tract, including the bladder.[4] Studies show that the risk for these cancers is independent of other factors like tobacco smoking, and these cancer rates are very high in persons who drink more than three cups of coffee a day. This risk is probably related to other compounds in coffee as well as caffeine.

It is well known that caffeine can cause damage to genetic material[5,6] and thereby can potentially lead to the development of cancer by altering DNA. It also interferes with the normal repair mechanisms of DNA and other genetic material. Caffeine can act as a teratogen, which is an agent that causes mistakes in gene production leading to malformations of a fetus.

Excessive coffee consumption by pregnant mothers can lead to lower birth weights of infants.[7] Pregnant women who consumed 600 mg or more of caffeine per day have a higher incidence of abortion and prematurity.[8] Both alcohol- and caffeine-containing products should be consumed in moderation.

11

Breast Cancer

ONE woman in eleven will develop breast cancer during her lifetime. It is the leading cause of death in women with cancer in the United States; 27 percent of the cancers that women develop are breast cancers. In 1983 in the United States, the new cases of breast cancer is about 114,900; 114,000 in women and 900 in men. Total deaths from breast cancer in 1983 are estimated to be 37,500; 37,200 females and 300 males. Black women are less likely to develop breast cancer than white women. However, black women have not done as well as white women once breast cancer has developed. This could be related to the extent of spread of the cancer (known as stage): it is usually more widespread in blacks than in whites at the time of diagnosis. Physicians use the term "stage of disease" to denote the extent to which a cancer has spread. The stage of breast cancer at diagnosis profoundly influences survival. There are three general terms to describe the stage: (1) localized—cancer is in its primary site of the breast; (2) regional—cancer has spread to lymph nodes in the region of the breast; and (3) distant—cancer has spread to other parts of the body. The prognosis worsens with each higher stage.

Breast cancer is more fatal in white men than in white women; of all those who survive for five years after the diagnosis has been made, 65 percent are women and 53 percent are men. This is because most people think that breast cancer is a woman's disease, and therefore when men get a lump in their breast or other symptoms related to their breasts, they tend to ignore it or dismiss it as not possibly being cancer. For all white breast cancer victims (both male and female) from 1960 to 1973, the length of time that most people survived from initial diagnosis was six years and seven months, compared to three years and eight months for blacks.[1] While several cancers, such as cancers of the uterus, stomach, liver, colon, and rectum, have decreased in women from 1930 to 1980, there has been little or no change in the death rate (survival rate) for breast cancer victims. For this very reason it is important to understand what role nutrition and other risk factors play in the development of breast cancer so that one can modify them accordingly wherever possible. An example of a risk factor that can be modified is a person's diet if it is high in animal fat. An example of a risk factor that cannot be modified is a person's genetic makeup (there are inherited risk factors which contribute to the development of breast cancer).

THE RISK FACTORS

Nutrition

Human breast cancer is associated with a high-fat diet, particularly animal fat.[2,3,4] Almost forty years ago A. Tannenbaum showed that dietary fat significantly favored the development and growth of both spontaneous and induced breast cancer in animals.[5] Since then, a high-animal-fat diet has been associated with human breast cancer, colon cancer, and coronary heart disease, suggesting that similar modifications of the diet will be beneficial in decreasing the risks of developing all these major diseases. Over the past half century the people of America have been consuming more fat, more cholesterol, more animal protein, more sugar, and less fiber and less starch. Likewise, there is a higher incidence of cancer and heart disease in the United States for the same time period.

Epidemiological studies are important to assess cancer trends. They show that there is a sixfold variation in breast cancer incidence in different parts of the world. High-risk countries like the United States are characterized by high standards of living with diets rich in cholesterol and animal fat. In high-risk countries there is a constant rate of increase in the rate of breast cancer development with age, but in low-risk countries the rate decreases after menopause.

Other epidemiological investigations have associated not only dietary fat but also total caloric intake (obesity) with the incidence of breast cancer.[6,7,8] Obesity seems to be a risk factor; breast cancer patients tend to be heavier and slightly taller than the average. Tannenbaum was one of the first investigators to show that the restriction of calories decreased the incidence of spontaneous breast cancers in mice. If calories were reduced by 30 percent from the carbohydrate fraction of the daily diet, cancer formation was inhibited.

A population of great interest in studying the incidence of breast cancer is the Seventh-Day Adventists in the United States. About half of them follow a vegetarian diet, and most do not eat pork. Breast cancer mortality is one half to two thirds of the breast cancer mortality seen in the general U.S. population.[9] R. L. Phillips has shown that the frequencies of eating five food items were associated with breast cancer: fried potatoes, hard fat (butter and margarine) for frying, all fried foods, some dairy products, and white bread. All these foods, except white bread, represent excellent sources of dietary fat.

In Japan, only 20 percent of the calories in the daily diet come from fat, compared to 40 percent in the United States. The incidence of colon and breast cancer is low in Japan and high in the United States. Japanese who come to the U.S. and adopt American customs and eating habits have the same incidence of colon cancer as Americans after living here for twenty years, and have the same incidence of breast cancer as Americans after only two generations.[10,11] Obviously nutrition is one major factor that accounts for these differences.

Another recent study shows that breast cancer mortality significantly correlates with an intestinal enzyme called lactase.[12] Lactase is responsible for the digestion of the milk sugar lactose. The enzyme is present in all mammals at birth and then starts to decrease after weaning, so that the adult human usually is incapable of digesting milk and many milk products. Exceptions to this pattern include populations of northwestern European origin (including the United States, Australia, and Canada), and scattered groups in other areas of the world in whom the enzyme is still present in varying amounts. These people historically consume a large amount of dairy products compared to other populations. Asians, Africans, and Mexicans, on the other hand, rarely have the enzyme lactase after childhood, and breast cancer mortality is only a small fraction of that seen in peoples who originate from northwestern Europe. This same study confirmed the findings of other investigations showing that breast cancer mortality is closely associated with the consumption of animal fat, milk, butter, and total calories.

Milk may be related to cancer in several ways. Milk consumption may contribute to the production of carcinogenic estrogens and other carcinogens by changing the type of bacteria in the intestine (more anaerobes) or by increasing the amount of cholesterol and bile acids available for the production of estrogens and other carcinogens. Also, it is known that mouse milk harbors a certain virus that can cause breast cancer in mice. When mouse milk is fed to baby mice, the cancer-producing virus is passed along and causes breast cancer. Milk from cows with leukemia harbors a cancer-producing virus which is infectious for several species. It is altogether possible, but not proven, that a cancer-producing virus in cow's milk may be passed along to humans who consume milk. Virus particles that can cause cancer have been found in human milk (see page 120). In addition, a person is exposed to other contaminants in milk. For example, DES (diethylstilbestrol) is used as a growth promoter for cattle. The amount of DES in milk is very small and probably cannot cause human breast cancer. However, there is no information concerning chronic low-level exposure to DES and its effect on cancer development. Additional contaminants that may inadvertently be included in milk are pesticides, industrial contaminants, and heavy metals.

A high-animal-fat diet can favor the development of breast cancer for many reasons. First, the typical high-fat American diet produces large amounts of sterol chemicals and bile acids in the intestine. Bacteria that normally live in our intestines can alter the sterol chemicals and bile acids produced by a high-fat diet in such a way to produce certain carcinogenic estrogens and other carcinogens affecting the breast.[13,14,15] This fact is supported by a great amount of research which has been reviewed by S. H. Brammer and colleagues.[16]

Second, large amounts of fatty tissue in the breasts may lead to greater amounts of estrogens in these tissues locally, which can be carcinogenic. An increased incidence of breast cancer is seen in heavier women who tend to have larger breasts and subsequently more fatty tissue in them.

Third, it has been shown that dietary polyunsaturated fats enhance cancer development. They do so more than saturated fats, presumably by increasing the hormone called prolactin.[17] A woman who eats a high-fat diet, especially high in unsaturated fats, has a very high blood prolactin level.[18] High prolactin levels are also found in women who have their first pregnancies late in life; this may account for the high risk for developing breast cancer seen in these women.

Polyunsaturated fats not only increase prolactin levels but can also be easily attacked by chemical-free radicals. As we discussed in Chapter 5, this is another mechanism by which polyunsaturated fats can lead to the development of cancer. Furthermore, polyunsaturated fatty acids in the serum may inhibit the normal function of the immune system and thus favor cancer development. And finally, the more polyunsaturated fats there are in cell membranes, the more susceptible the cell is to carcinogenic agents.

Substances in breast fluid may also have an influence on the development of breast cancer. Breast fluid secretion occurs in most women, but in varying amounts. For example, Oriental women have much less breast fluid secretion than white women, and they also have a lower incidence of breast cancer. Breast fluid bathes the ductal cells of the breast gland. Many of the breast cancers originate in the ductal cells of the gland, so the fluid that bathes the cells may have an effect on the development of cancer. A study involving 252 Finnish women revealed that about one third of them had very high prolactin levels in their breast fluid compared to their blood. However, this study by P. Hill has not yet been extended for a long enough period of time to determine whether this group will eventually develop breast cancer. The prolactin content of breast fluid from Oriental women has not yet been determined, so no conclusion can be made concerning breast fluid prolactin level and its effect on the development of breast cancer.

A chemical substance derived from cholesterol called cholesterol epoxide has been found in human breast fluid.[19] The higher the blood cholesterol level the higher the cholesterol epoxide level in breast fluid. Cholesterol epoxide is a carcinogen for animals. The potential of its acting as a carcinogen in humans is very real. Hence, this is another reason to keep your blood cholesterol level low—so that your breast fluid level of cholesterol epoxide is also low and lessens the potential risk of cancer development.

Nicotine and its close relative cotinine have been shown to appear in breast fluid within five minutes after smoking.[20]

So far no studies have shown a conclusive relationship between smoking and the development of breast cancer. However, it is well known that there are fifteen carcinogens derived from smoking. And the fact that nicotine can be detected in breast fluid indicates that many other environmental factors may be present, many of which may be carcinogenic. Chemicals may be held in breast fluid longer than in the blood because there are more lipids inside the breast. Therefore, known risk factors for cancer in general, such as tobacco smoking, should be eliminated altogether because carcinogens get into breast fluid, bathe breast tissue for long periods of time, and may lead to the development of cancer.

Trauma

Perhaps one of the worst misconceptions about the development of breast cancer is trauma. Trauma, such as a bump into the car steering wheel or a blow to the breast, will not cause breast cancer. Likewise, fondling or caressing the breast will not cause breast cancer.

Age

Age is a risk factor for breast cancer. Generally, the longer an individual lives the more likely it is that the person will develop cancer. The incidence of breast cancer rises rapidly when a woman enters her forties, levels off between forty-five and fifty-five, then rises again more slowly during the postmenopausal years. Age is a risk factor that one can do little about.

Family History of Breast Cancer

If a woman has had breast cancer once, she has an increased risk for developing cancer again, either in the same breast or in the opposite breast. Ten to 25 percent of women with breast cancer in one breast also have it in the other. There is a two- to threefold increased risk for developing breast cancer in women who have a sister or mother diagnosed with breast cancer.

Hormonal Factors

A woman's reproductive history can be another risk factor. Women with a long menstrual history, characterized by beginning menstrual cycles early in life and starting menopause very late in life, are at an increased risk for developing breast cancer when compared to others. Women are less at risk for developing breast cancer if they have had a natural early menopause, or if they have had their ovaries removed and hence had an early menopause artificially. The older a woman is at the time of her first pregnancy the higher is her risk for developing breast cancer. A woman who delivers her first child after the age of 35 has a threefold higher risk for breast cancer than a woman who bears her first child before the age of 18. The number of pregnancies does not seem to have much effect on the risk. Women who have never been pregnant have the same risk as women who became pregnant late in life.

Fibrocystic breast disease, a benign disorder that affects almost 50 percent of all women during some time of their lives, is a risk factor for breast cancer. This increased risk persists for as long as thirty years after diagnosis has been made. The more abnormal and the more enlarged (atypia and hyperplasia) the fibrocystic breast cells are at the time of diagnosis, the higher the risk of developing breast cancer in the future. As was discussed in Chapter 6, vitamin E might have a role in the treatment of fibrocystic breast disease.

Exogenous estrogens (estrogens taken by mouth) affect some cells' division and may make them abnormal. Normally the hormones produced by the body are in a very delicate balance. If additional hormones are taken by a person, the tissues that respond to them may become abnormal and cancerous. In an extensive review of the literature it was shown that estrogens taken by mouth increase the risk of cancer of the endometrium (uterus lining).[21] In addition to an increased risk for developing cancer of the endometrium, exogenous estrogens are also implicated in an increased incidence of breast cancer. Exogenous estrogens administered in large amounts have been associated with breast cancer in male transsexuals[22,23,24] as well as in male heart and ulcer patients.[25,26] The use of estrogens by postmenopausal women to relieve menopausal symptoms seems to increase the risk of developing breast cancer in these women;[27,28,29] some other studies show no such effect, however.

A subject of great controversy is whether oral contraceptives can cause breast cancer. Several very compelling and clear studies show that oral contraceptives do cause an increase in the incidence of breast cancer in women regardless of whether they have had benign cystic breast disease or not,[30,31,32,33] although other studies show no increased risk. The study by M. C. Pike and colleagues also showed that a first-trimester abortion before a first full-term pregnancy causes a substantial increase in risk of developing breast cancer.[34] The controversy about whether the Pill causes breast cancer will probably continue for some years, but current evidence indicates that it does cause an increased risk. And the United States Food and Drug Administration now requires that package inserts of oral contraceptives warn consumers of the suspected link to breast cancer.[35]

Approximately 2 million women took DES (diethylstilbestrol) to avert miscarriages in the 1940s and 1950s. These women and their children add up to about 4 to 6 million people exposed to DES. There is ample evidence now which indicates that daughters of women who were exposed to DES have a higher incidence of cancer of the vagina, cervix, endometrium, and breast. Sons of DES-exposed mothers may have reproductive and urinary tract abnormalities. One of these abnormalities in men is undescended testicles, which if uncorrected before the age of 6, is a risk factor for developing cancer of the testicles. This information is derived from a recent study which compiled data from 1950 to 1952 concerning mothers who were in a randomized clinical trial—50 percent were given DES and 50 percent were given a placebo (reported by the National Cancer Institute in *The Breast Cancer Digest* in December 1979). Besides informing your physician, the following are recommendations by the research task force for women who were exposed to DES.

1. Tell your daughter or son about your DES exposure.
2. Try to obtain the details of your DES dosage and the duration you took it.
3. Have an annual physical examination (the same type of examination all women should have if they are over 20, or younger if they are sexually active). The examination should include:
   a. A pelvic examination with a Pap smear;
   b. A breast examination by a physician;
   c. Mammography (X-ray study of the breast) under the following conditions if you have no symptoms of breast cancer:
      (1) No mammography under the age of 35
      (2) Mammography if you are between 35 and 39 and have already had breast cancer
      (3) Mammography if you are between 40 and 49 and have a personal history of breast cancer or have a close relative with a history of breast cancer
      (4) Mammography possibly annually if you are over 50
4. Practice breast self-examination every month. Report anything suspicious to your doctor. Eighty percent of all breast lumps are not cancer, however.
5. Report any unusual bleeding or discharge from the vagina to a physician immediately.
6. Avoid exposure to other estrogens. This includes oral contraceptives, estrogens as a "morning-after" pill, and estro-

gens used as replacement therapy during or after menopause.

The recommendations for a daughter of a DES-exposed mother are similar:

1. If unusual bleeding or discharge occurs from the vagina at any age see your physician immediately.
2. If you have no symptoms you should have a pelvic examination including a Pap smear at least once a year starting at age 14 or when you begin to menstruate—whichever is first.
3. During the pelvic exam, the vaginal walls should be temporarily stained so the physician can see any abnormalities.
4. Follow-up examinations are most important.

The recommendations for sons of DES-exposed mothers are that they should see a physician to check their reproductive and urinary systems to make certain there are no abnormalities.

Radiation

Radiation exposure is another risk factor for breast cancer. An increased number of breast cancer cases was found in Japanese people who were exposed to radiation in the bombing of Hiroshima. Women with tuberculosis who had multiple chest X-rays following treatment had substantially increased incidence of breast cancer.

Viruses

There is no evidence thus far incriminating viruses as the cause of human cancer. There are several animal models which show conclusively that some viruses cause cancer, especially in mice. Virus particles similar to the mouse breast cancer virus have been found in human breast milk. It appears that these virus particles may be more prevalent in women who have a family history of breast cancer. These virus particles have been detected frequently in Parsi women, a group in India which has a very high incidence of breast cancer. I'm sure that eventually there will be conclusive evidence showing that viruses do cause some human cancers. A normally functioning immune system, plus good nutrition with the proper vitamins and minerals will in part safeguard against viruses and other dietary risk factors.

PREVENTIVE MEASURES

Having any or all of the risk factors does not necessarily mean that a woman will actually develop breast cancer. However, women who are included in any of the three major risk categories should practice breast self-examination and should consider other detection techniques such as mammography according to the criteria already discussed. The three major risk groups are:

1. Advanced age
2. Previous personal history of breast cancer
3. Mother or sister who had breast cancer

The following categories are also risk factors for developing breast cancer:

1. High dietary intake of animal fat
2. Obesity
3. History of breast cancer in your grandmother or aunt (father's or mother's sister)
4. History of fibrocystic breast disease
5. First baby born after age 30
6. Never been pregnant
7. Abortion in first trimester before ever having a full-term pregnancy
8. Early start of menses and late onset of menopause
9. Excessive exposure to radiation
10. History of cancer of the endometrium, ovary, or colon
11. Estrogen therapy for menopause or birth control (oral contraceptives)

Breast Cancer Detection

Since breast cancer mortality is directly related to how extensive the disease is at time of diagnosis, it seems reasonable then to advocate methods of early detection. One such method, breast self-examination, can be performed by every woman after being properly taught. About 90 percent of breast cancer symptoms are found by women themselves, either accidentally or by self-examination. Although 96 percent of women surveyed by the National Cancer Institute were aware of breast self-examination, only 40 percent actually did it. It is important to learn this technique properly, otherwise a woman who examines her breasts incorrectly may have a false sense of security when she finds no masses. A recent study revealed that only 20 percent of women (161 in the group studied by H. Howe) were proficient at detecting about half of the lumps in a model of a breast with seven lumps in it. As you can tell from this, a woman who actually goes through the motions of breast self-examination every month may not be able to find the cancer mass in her breast. Therefore breast examinations should be done in conjunction with a yearly physical examination by a qualified physician.

Breast self-examination should be done a few days after your menstrual period because your breasts are not swollen or tender at that time. After menopause you should pick a particular day each month, like the first Monday of the month, to examine your breasts.

The first step in breast self-examination is to stand in front of the mirror without clothing from your waist up. You must look for any changes in the shape or size of your breasts, for discharge from the nipples, for pulling inward of the nipples, or changes in the appearance of the skin, like dimpling or an orange-peel appearance. Since changes in the breast may be accentuated by changing the position of your body and arms, you should lean forward next and observe; then put your hands behind your head and observe; and finally, observe after you place your hands on your hips, pushing inward on your hips with your hands.

The next few steps begin by lying on your back and placing a folded towel under your right shoulder first. The towel acts to raise the breast and allows for easier examination. Now put your right hand and arm behind your head. With your left hand, move your fingers in a circular motion around your breast, working in from the outer edge of the breast to the nipple, in order to explore for masses. Do not pinch your breast between your thumb and fingers because this may give you the false impression of a mass. Feel gently but firmly. Thoroughly examine the area between your breast and axilla (armpit), because this is the location of some of the lymph nodes that drain the breast. Repeat the process now on the opposite side.

If you think anything is abnormal, contact your physician. You can write to the National Cancer Institute in Bethesda, Maryland, for information on free classes in your area about breast self-examination, or call toll-free 800–638–6694.

Mammography is a sensitive X-ray technique that helps to detect breast masses. The current National Cancer Institute criteria for using mammography have already been outlined in this chapter.

A woman with one or more of the risk factors for breast cancer should probably be seen by a physician twice a year, have a mammography if indicated according to the accepted criteria, and perform monthly breast self-examinations. If a woman has none of the risk factors for breast cancer, she should practice breast self-examination monthly, have a physical examination yearly, and obtain a mammography according to the criteria already outlined.

In this chapter we have examined the risk factors associated with breast cancer. Some of them can be modified and others cannot. Nutrition appears to play an important role, and these dietary factors (high animal fat, obesity, etc.) should be eliminated or modified substantially to reduce the associated risk. By modifying all the risk factors that you can, you lessen your overall risk of developing this number-one female cancer killer. It is just good common sense!

12

Gastrointestinal and Other Cancers

GASTROINTESTINAL cancers are the second leading cause of death among all cancer victims. The death rate for cancer of the colon and rectum has been about the same for the past half century. Death due to cancer of the pancreas has increased slightly, while the mortality rate from stomach cancer has decreased substantially over this same period for both men and women. The total number of new gastrointestinal cancer cases estimated for 1983 was 202,400; the total number of deaths from gastrointestinal cancer is about 115,200. Nutrition appears to play a dominant role in this group of cancers.

COLON AND RECTAL CANCER

Together, colon and rectal cancers are the most frequently diagnosed cancers in the United States with the exception of skin cancer. Because of this, it is important to make an early diagnosis, and even more important to eliminate all known risk factors. A major risk factor involved in the development of colon/rectal cancer is the food that you eat. Meat, cholesterol, animal fat, and low fiber consumption are very closely correlated with the development of colon cancer.

There are major differences in death rates from colon cancer

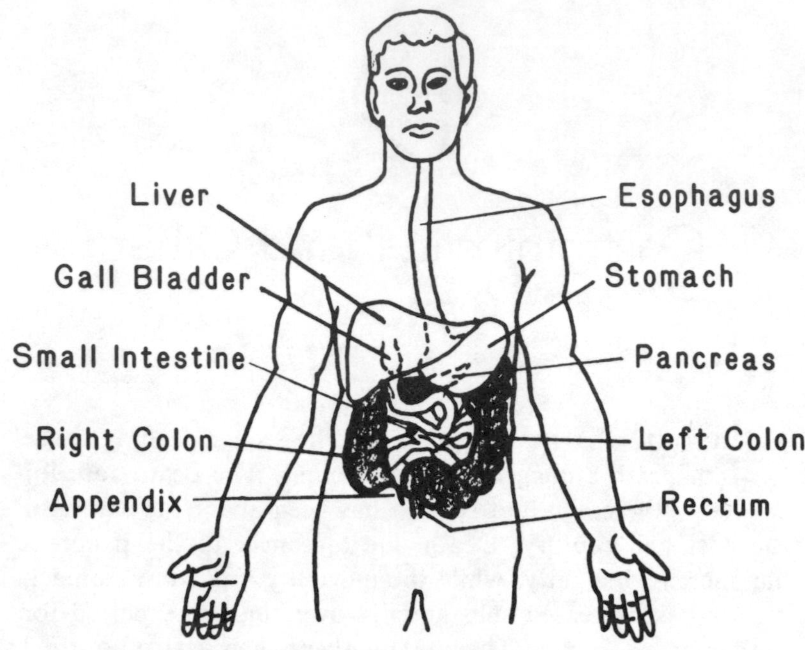

Figure 4. Representation of the Gastrointestinal Tract

in different parts of the world, and epidemiological studies show that dietary factors account for the different incidence rates. The more industrialized a country, the higher the rate of colon cancer (two exceptions are Japan and Finland), because the people in an industrialized country usually eat more animal fat, beef, and cholesterol-containing foods than do people in nonindustrialized countries. The highest colon cancer incidence rates are found in Western Europe and in English-speaking countries; the lowest incidence rates are found in Asia, Africa, and South America (with the exception of Uruguay and Argentina, where the rates are similar to those of North America). In countries with a high incidence of colon cancer most of the cancers are located in the left colon and rectum, whereas in countries with a low incidence most of the cancers are in the right colon. Dr. Dennis Burkitt offers the following analogy for this distribution of cancer since carcinogens become progressively more concentrated at the end of the gastrointestinal tract (left colon and rectum). While a man proceeds down a path carrying a leaky pot of water containing a tablet of dye which is gradually dissolving, the water becomes more deeply colored because: (1) the volume will be progressively reduced and the dye more concentrated, and (2) more dye will be progressively dissolved.

If persons emigrate from a country with a low incidence rate of colon cancer to a country with a high rate, the higher cancer rate shows up within the first generation. Before World War II, the Japanese got the bulk of their calories from rice, and the incidence of colon cancer was then very low. Among the Japanese who immigrated to Hawaii and California after the war, a significant increase of colon cancer was seen in the first generation and more particularly in the second generation. The main reason for this was the consumption of Western foods such as milk, eggs, and beef. The incidence of colon cancer is rising now in Japan, especially among young Japanese whose diets are more like diets of the West.

A population group at high risk for developing colon/rectal cancer is American-born Jews of European descent living in Israel. However, a twenty-year study has shown that a diet high in fiber, with polyunsaturated fats and supplemented with vitamin C, substantially reduces the number of colon/rectal cancer cases in this group.[1] Seventh-Day Adventists and Mormons have a substantially lesser incidence of colon cancer than the general population.[2,3] Both groups consume a lot of dietary fiber and little or no beef and animal fat. People in Finland have a low incidence of colon cancer, but they have a high fat intake. However, the bulk of their fat calories are derived from dairy products rather than beef. They also consume a great amount of fiber in their diet, which may play a protective role. Other studies also suggest that a high intake of animal fat, beef, and low dietary fiber have a strong association with colon cancer.[4,5,6,7] Beef is a high-fat meat contributing about 40 percent of the total fat calories in the American population. People who consume large amounts of animal fat usually eat very little fiber.

How do meat, animal fat, cholesterol, and low fiber in one's diet relate to the development of colon cancer? The answers are to be found in the contents of the colon itself. The intestine is lined with billions of various bacteria that help to digest our food, produce certain vitamins, and perform several other functions. There are two main groups of bacteria: those that need oxygen to live, called aerobes, and those that do not need oxygen, called anaerobes. It is known that what one eats greatly influences the type of bacteria in the intestine. Dietary fat determines the amount of acid and neutral sterol chemicals in the colon as well as the type of bacteria that acts on those chemicals.

As was suggested in Chapter 7, carcinogens and cocarcinogens may exist in food products. Fungus and its possible toxic substances were also mentioned. Bacteria and their products are yet another source of potential carcinogens and cocarcinogens, which are formed by bacteria from acid and neutral sterol chemicals in the colon.[8] Some bacterial products include actinomycin D and mitomycin C, potential carcinogens, and streptozotocin, which causes cancer of the renal cortex of the kidney.[9]

Stools from persons in the United States and Britain, where the incidence of colon cancer is very high, have much higher counts of anaerobic bacteria (non–oxygen users) than those from people in Uganda or South India, where the incidence of the disease is low. In another study, the International Agency for Research on Cancer found in 1977 that Danes in Copenhagen had ten times more anaerobic bacteria and a higher incidence of colon cancer than Finns in Kuopio, who have a low incidence of colon cancer and ten times less anaerobic bacteria in their colon.

Dietary animal fat substantially increases the number of anaerobic bacteria, which produce carcinogens. B. Maier et al. found that ten American students who ate absolutely no meat for four weeks had a very high amount of aerobic bacteria and lower levels of anaerobic bacteria. When the same students were fed meat, many more anaerobic bacteria grew.[10] Certain strains of an anaerobic bacteria called clostridia are capable of producing carcinogens from bile acids. An experiment using rats showed that if one group of rats was fed dietary fatty foods and also had all their gastrointestinal bacteria eliminated, the incidence of gastrointestinal cancer was much lower than the incidence of cancers seen in animals which were fed the same dietary fat but retained their gut bacteria.[11] Together, the dietary animal fat and anaerobic bacteria, which produce carcinogens and other chemicals, develop more colon cancer than just the dietary fat alone. It seems prudent therefore to decrease or eliminate beef and other sources of dietary animal fat so that the number of anaerobic bacteria is kept normal and thereby decrease one's risk for developing colon cancer.

It is also known that certain enzymes are made by bacteria in response to dietary beef and animal fat. These enzymes are made to aid in the digestion of beef, but they also can convert cocarcinogens into carcinogens. These enzymes include nitrosoreductase, azoreductase, and beta-glucuronidase.

Dietary animal fats also increase bile acid production; bile acids are excreted from the gallbladder into the gastrointestinal tract. They get mixed with the stools and travel along the colon where they are converted into carcinogens and cocarcinogens by colonic bacteria.[12,13,14,15,16] The more beef and animal fat you eat, the greater the potential for the production of more carcinogens in the colon.

A certain amount of time is required by the colon bacteria

to convert bowel contents into carcinogens. The longer the stools stay in the colon, the greater the potential for an increased production of carcinogens and their buildup. And the longer the carcinogens touch the inside of the colon, the greater the risk for the development of colon cancer. Hence, a more rapid transit time should be associated with a decreased risk of developing colon cancer. Transit time is the amount of time required by food to travel through the gastrointestinal tract from the mouth to the anus.

People in agricultural societies have a rapid transit time. Several studies have shown that a rapid transit time, which is associated with a diet high in indigestible fiber, is protective against the development of colon cancer.[17,18] Another study supporting this finding involves the epidemiological investigation of Finns and Americans in New York City.[19] Finns in Kuopio, Finland, are a low-risk population for the development of colon cancer, and North Americans are a high-risk group. The major part of the Finns' dietary fat comes from milk and other dairy products, whereas the major source of dietary fat for Americans is beef and animal fat. Finns consume low amounts of meat and high amounts of cereal compared to Americans. The daily output of stools (by weight) is three times greater by Finns than by Americans. Bile acids, carcinogens, and carcinogen-producing enzymes were detected in both groups' stools, but much less so in the stools of the Finns because the great volume of their daily stools simply dilutes all the carcinogens (and those carcinogens that are there are moved out of the colon much more quickly). Hence, both the large volume of the stool and the increased transit time contribute to the Finns' decreased risk of colon cancer.

Fiber

Fiber is a complex carbohydrate consisting of a polysaccharide and a lignin substance that provides the structure of the plant cell. It is undigested residue that reaches the end of the small intestine. There are three groups of dietary fiber types: (1) vegetable fibers, which are highly fermentable and have a low undigested content; (2) bran, which is less fermentable; and (3) purified fibers such as cellulose, which are much less fermentable and have a high undigested content.

Recently the subject of dietary fiber has been reviewed extensively.[20] This complex substance can act as a "glue" for certain chemicals. For instance, unconjugated bile acids which are produced by the body can be adsorbed to fiber in the colon and passed out in the stool without intestinal bacteria forming carcinogens from those bile acids.[21] In addition some fiber binds to cholesterol and lipids, nitrogen, and certain minerals, and eliminates them in the stool. This action in essence lowers the blood concentration of cholesterol and certain other lipids, nitrogen; and some minerals such as zinc, calcium, and iron.[22] (The effects of fiber on cholesterol and lipids will be discussed in Chapter 13.) Also, B. H. Ershoff has shown that various poisons added to food can be neutralized if fiber-rich foods are eaten.[23] Fiber holds a great deal of water and this is responsible for the increased weight and amount of stool excreted every day. If 16 grams of cellulose or bran is added to a normal diet every day, stool weight will almost double because of the increased water content. Moreover, without fiber, solids move down the tract more slowly than water and that is the common problem in people who have diverticular disease.

George Oettle in 1960 was the first person to associate dietary fiber consumption with a low risk of developing colon cancer. He noted that the Bantu tribe, living in the rural areas of South Africa, had a very low incidence of colon cancer. Also, they excreted large piles of feces, which was related to the great amount of fiber they ate. Another student of Africa, Dennis Burkitt, wrote about Oettle's observation. Burkitt stated that a high-fiber diet results in a rapid transit time for solid material to pass through the gastrointestinal tract and also increases the amount of stool. And these two variables are associated with a decreased risk of colon cancer as described by Oettle, Burkitt, and others.[24,25,26,27,28,29,30,31] Diet in rural Africa and in other similar locations provides about 25 grams of crude fiber daily, whereas Western diets provide less than 5 grams of fiber daily. Patients who have diverticular disease consume about 3.5 grams of fiber per day.[32] With a more rapid transit time, bile acids and other carcinogens produced by anaerobic intestinal bacteria (fostered by dietary fat) move out of the gastrointestinal tract more quickly. Furthermore, since the volume of feces is increased, those carcinogens that are produced pass through the gut more diluted. Hence, if more dietary fiber is eaten, carcinogens pass out of the gut more quickly and there are fewer carcinogens per square inch.

Table I in Chapter 16 lists various foods and their fiber content. Bran, carrots, oranges, apples (pectin), brussels sprouts, and cabbage are the best fiber sources that bind water. Alfalfa, wheat straw, and some other fibers bind considerable amounts of bile acids which otherwise could promote colon cancer.[33] Chlorophyll was recently shown to be the major factor in wheat sprout that inhibits carcinogens which require metabolic activation.[34]

Besides colon cancer, some studies reviewed by Burkitt postulate that dietary fiber may play a protective role in diverticular disease, diabetes, heart disease, obesity, gallbladder disease, and peptic ulcer disease.[35,36] Future studies need to be carried out using standard types of fiber so that results of the studies will be more meaningful.

Other Risk Factors for Colon Cancer

Other risk factors for colon/rectal cancer include:

1. Familial polyposis—multiple polyps in the colon
2. Ulcerative colitis (inflammation of the colon) for more than ten years
3. Gardner's syndrome

4. Elevated intake of calories, total protein, and cholesterol[37]
5. Asbestos exposure

Colon Cancer Detection

Screening for colon cancer in persons 40 years old or older who have no symptoms whatsoever should include an annual physical examination with a rectal exam and a stool examination for traces of blood. Blood in the stool, unnoticed by the eye, may be an early warning signal for an otherwise undetected colon cancer. In this situation, the stool would look normal to you if there were only traces of blood in it. In addition, you should have a sigmoidoscopy done. A sigmoidoscope is a tubelike device 25 centimeters long with a light on the end. It is placed in the anus by a physician as far as its length. The physician can then directly visualize the rectum and a portion of the sigmoid colon. Fifty-five percent of all large-bowel cancers occur in this very short segment of the colon (25 centimeters). Therefore, if this area is routinely checked and a cancer is detected in a person who has no symptoms, therapy can begin sooner. Removal of all polyps detected by sigmoidoscopy sharply reduces the incidence of cancer in this area of the colon.[38,39]

For persons with a high risk of developing colon/rectal cancer, a sigmoidoscopy should be done annually. High-risk patients include those whose diets are high in beef, animal fat, cholesterol, and low in fiber, and those who have the risk factors listed above. Persons 40 years old or older who are not at high risk and who have no symptoms, should have a sigmoidoscopy every two years or so.[40]

MOUTH AND ESOPHAGUS CANCER

An association has been made between the Plummer-Vinson syndrome (anemia and epithelial lesions) and cancer of the mouth (hypopharynx) in Swedish women. Iron deficiency, as well as some vitamin deficiencies, may be responsible for this syndrome.[41] Improved nutrition and health care lead to a decreased incidence of the syndrome and cancer.[42] Other risk factors associated with the development of cancer of the mouth and pharynx are alcohol, tobacco, and nutritional deficiencies. There is a precancerous lesion which can be found in the mouth, called leukoplakia—a thin white area of mucosa that cannot be rubbed off. This should be biopsied and followed by a physician.

The incidence of cancer of the esophagus differs greatly in different parts of the world by as much as a factor of 500. Soviet Central Asia, northern Iran, northern China, and southern and eastern Africa have the highest incidence of esophageal cancer. Curiously, less than 500 miles from each of these areas is an area of low or moderate incidence of esophageal cancer.

There are several major risk factors for the development of esophageal cancer. Smoking tobacco and excessive alcohol consumption are two main risk factors in the United States, Brittany, and Normandy. However, there are areas of the world which have high incidence of esophageal cancer and where the use of alcohol is forbidden by religious teachings. Tobacco contains 16 known carcinogens. A recent study by T. Hirayama showed that people who both drank and smoked every day had five times the normal rate of cancers of the mouth cavity and three times the rate for esophageal cancer. All alcoholic beverages increased the number of cancer cases of the esophagus, but different percentages of alcohol content produced different cancer incidence rates. For example, beer drinkers had the lowest rate of esophageal cancers compared to the other alcohol consumers. The risk increases with saki and then whiskey. In addition the study shows that bracken fern, a plant from certain areas of the world, when eaten by humans is a risk factor for esophageal cancer.[43]

Another risk factor is long-term irritation of the esophageal mucosa (cells which line the inner surface of the esophagus on which food passes to the stomach). Swallowing lye is one such irritation that can lead to the development of esophageal cancer. Carcinogens which may be in foods or which are the result of food processing or cooking can also adversely act on the esophageal mucosa.

STOMACH CANCER

For the past fifty years the number of new cases and of deaths from stomach cancer has been decreasing steadily, so that now deaths are only 25 percent of what they were in 1930. One of the reasons for this is probably the accessibility and widespread use of refrigeration today, lower consumption of smoked foods, increased consumption of green vegetables and fruit, and reduction in use of salt pickling. (Pickled fish contain carcinogens which act on the stomach.) Prior to refrigeration, meats and fish were preserved with nitrates, which could be converted to nitrites at room temperature. The nitrites then form the very potent carcinogens nitrosamines, which were probably responsible for the huge number of stomach cancers before refrigeration. With the advent of refrigeration, there was no longer the need for the great use of nitrites as preservatives. Hence, the number of people developing stomach cancer dropped dramatically. Nitrites are still used in some bacons, hot dogs, and other foods.

Read the label on foods! Nitrates are used in fertilizers and are ingested in the agricultural products that we eat. Nitrates are converted into nitrites by saliva and intestinal bacteria. A few vegetables contain some nitrates.[44] Those with the greatest amounts of nitrates are beets, squash, parsley, turnips, radishes, celery, cabbage, lettuce, spinach, string beans, and eggplant.[45] The change from nitrate to nitrite is prevented by vitamin C, and this vitamin is found in all plants. However, we can avoid non–agriculturally grown nitrite-containing foods such as bacon and hot dogs. And in addition, we can consume more vitamin C since vitamin C inhibits the formation of nitrosamines. The vitamin C content in a balanced Western diet is nutritionally sufficient, but is insufficient to inhibit the formation of nitrosamines.[46]

Diet is reported to be a significant risk factor for stomach cancer, especially in the Japanese, where a study found significant deficiencies in vitamin A and calcium as well as relative deficiencies in consumption of green and yellow vegetables.[47] Vitamin A, found in those vegetables, has anticancer effects. Diet is the major risk factor for stomach cancer in people in Minnesota, Wisconsin, and northern Michigan. The hypothesis is that these people have assimilated their diets with the diets of immigrants from Finland, Poland, Norway, and Sweden, who have high stomach cancer rates.[48] The specific dietary factors there have not yet been identified, but high carbohydrate consumption, low consumption of fresh fruits and vegetables, and high amount of nitrites constitute the major dietary risk factors for stomach cancer as determined in another study.[49]

Another risk factor in the development of stomach cancer is smoking. Also, asbestos exposure is a risk factor for cancer in the gastrointestinal organs, especially the stomach.

LIVER CANCER

Liver cancer is a major problem in many parts of the world. Areas of Africa have high rates of liver cancer, and several studies have observed a relationship between children with enlarged livers due to malnutrition and liver cancer. There is a high frequency of liver cancer in Africa associated with coexisting cirrhosis. Vitamin deficiencies, particularly the B vitamins, are yet another risk factor.[50] Alcohol is also a risk factor for liver cancer.

Aflatoxin, a potent carcinogen derived from plants, especially peanut plants, probably directly causes human liver cancer, although conclusive evidence is not yet available. Today in the U.S. batches of peanuts must be assayed for aflatoxin before they are sold to processors.

Many people in Asia and Africa get viral hepatitis early in life. These people have a very high rate of liver cancer. The virus responsible for hepatitis may also transform the liver cells into cancer cells. Having viral hepatitis may be a risk factor for liver cancer years after the initial infection.

Hormones as risk factors for liver cancer have already been discussed in Chapter 2.

GALLBLADDER CANCER

Cancer of the gallbladder and its ducts causes eighty deaths per week in the United States. Gallstones are the major known cause of gallbladder cancer. This is probably because the stones are a constant source of irritation to the inside of the gallbladder. Any time there is a constant irritation of a tissue, the potential for developing a cancer is high. Therefore it becomes important to know all the risk factors that predispose to gallstones, since these risk factors are really the same for gallbladder cancer. The risk factors include being female, age over 45, women who are still fertile, estrogen therapy (birth control pills, etc.), obesity, and elevated cholesterol and other lipids. Do these risk factors sound familiar by now? Mexican-Americans, Indians of the southwest, and whites of Appalachia have these risk factors and have a high incidence of gallstones and a higher than normal incidence of gallbladder cancer.

To safeguard against the potential of developing gallbladder cancer one must modify the known risk factors. The diet should be appropriately modified by reducing cholesterol-containing foods, eliminating animal fat, avoiding estrogens, and reducing your weight if you are obese. Patients with gallbladders loaded with calcified gallstones should have the gallbladder removed if they are in good physical condition, because the risk of developing gallbladder cancer is very high, varying from 12 to 62 percent depending on what study you read.[51]

In some parts of the world, parasite infections of the gall bladder and ducts are thought to be responsible for causing gallbladder cancer: liver-flukes in the Orient, *Clonorchis sinensis* and *Opisthorchis felineus* in Asia, and *O. viverrini* in Thailand and Malaysia. The diet of Thais contains a great deal of nitrosamines, the potent carcinogen. This may help promote cancer in a gallbladder that has already been assaulted by a parasitic infection.

There may be carcinogens that affect workers in rubber plants and automotive plants, since there is a higher incidence of gallbladder cancer in these workers than in the normal population.[52] However, the specific carcinogen(s) have not yet been identified.

PANCREAS CANCER

Cancer of the pancreas has been steadily increasing since 1930. It is the fourth most common fatal cancer in the United States. There are about 22,600 estimated deaths in 1983 from pancreatic cancer, far more than deaths from either stomach cancer, esophageal cancer, or small-intestine cancer. The reasons for this are unclear, but excessive alcohol consumption throughout life is an important risk factor. Many alcoholics at one time or another have had pancreatitis (inflammation of the pancreas) resulting from alcohol. When the pancreas tries to heal itself after repeated assaults, abnormal cells could result and lead to the development of cancer. Other investigators feel differently, however.

Poor dietary factors have been implicated as a risk factor for pancreas cancer, particularly a high-fat diet.[53] This is certainly true of alcoholics who live on alcohol as their only source of calories. Smoking is also a risk factor, a fact which is very consistent in many studies.

A recent study shows that drinking coffee may also be a risk factor for pancreatic cancer.[54] The study shows that drinking two cups of coffee every day increases the risk of developing pancreatic cancer by a factor of 1.8, and drinking three or more cups daily increases the risk to 2.7 times the rate seen in the normal population. It is a little premature to say that coffee consumption is a risk factor for the development of pancreatic cancer, since considerable doubt has been cast upon this study.[55,56] However, Seventh-Day Adventists and Mormons, who do not consume caffeine, have very low rates of pancreatic cancer. But these groups do not drink alcohol or smoke, either.

OTHER CANCERS

Prostate

In 1983, an estimated 24,100 men will die of prostate cancer. The death rate is higher in American blacks than American whites, and even higher than the death rate seen in blacks in Nigeria. Nutrition and hormones seem to be risk factors in this cancer.

There is a four- to fivefold increased risk for the development of prostate cancer in men who have enlarged prostates, a condition known as benign prostatic hypertrophy.[57] This benign condition is very common in older men and may be the result of a high-cholesterol, high-fat diet. Cancer of the prostate is higher in immigrant Japanese living in Hawaii than in Japanese living in Japan. A major difference between the two groups is the diet, the former group eating an "American" diet which is high in animal fat and cholesterol.

After age 50 male hormones start to decrease. But in many

men with prostate cancers, testosterone levels are the same as the levels seen in men with benign prostatic hypertrophy. The continued presence of the hormone may also be an activating factor for prostate cancer. Receiving testosterone injections to restore or rejuvenate potency in older men who have become impotent due to low hormone levels may be dangerous, because testosterone could activate a dormant prostatic cancer.

Endometrial Cancer

Endometrial cancer is a cancer of the inner lining of the uterus. Obesity has been reported to be a risk factor.[58] There is excellent correlation to show that high dietary fat is another risk factor for endometrial cancer.[59]

This cancer is seen in women who begin menstrual periods early in life and have a later onset of menopause; their endometrium has been stimulated with hormones for a very long time. The incidence of this cancer has been increasing over the past fifteen years, which could be related to the increased usage of estrogens for birth control and for symptoms of menopause.

Urinary Bladder Cancer

In 1895 a German urologist named L. Rehn observed a relationship between urinary bladder cancer and certain dyes in industry. Presently about 20 percent of bladder cancers can be attributed to chemicals in industry. Beta-naphthylamine was the first chemical found to produce human bladder cancer. Compounds with aromatic amines have been implicated as well.

In 1950 dietary tryptophan and its breakdown products were found to be a risk factor for bladder cancer.[60] Tryptophan-rich foods include cow's milk, human milk, wheat (white flour), maize, beef, and eggs. Since then other dietary risk factors have been found. In 1977 there was a flurry of reports concerning artificial sweeteners as risk factors for bladder cancer. Other more recent studies show that artificial sweeteners pose no increased risk for bladder cancer.[61,62] A similar story is seen with cyclamate use. The implication of coffee as a bladder carcinogen was made while A. B. Miller was studying bladder cancer patients.[63] However, there is not enough conclusive evidence to point to coffee as a risk factor yet.

Bracken fern (*Pteridium aquilinum*) is a naturally occurring bladder carcinogen. This plant is eaten by cattle in certain parts of the world and the cattle develop bladder cancer. This carcinogen is found in cow's milk which is drunk by humans there. So far no increased evidence of bladder cancer is reported, but these people do have a much higher rate of esophageal cancer.[64]

Since the bladder's function is to hold water for long periods of time, any carcinogens that do get into the urine will also affect the bladder wall. Investigators are now looking at the nitrate and nitrite content of the water we drink, which can form nitrosamine. It has already been reported that some bladder cancer patients have high levels of N-butyl-N-(hydroxybutyl) nitrosamine but it has not yet been established whether this chemical has come from the water supply. Other risk factors for bladder cancer are smoking and a high-animal-fat diet.[65,66]

There are several protective measures one can take. Obviously, the first thing to do is to eliminate the risk factors. Also, 25 mg of pyridoxine (vitamin B_6) per day can decrease the risk of tryptophan's effects[67] and diminish the frequency of "recurring" bladder cancers.[68] Finally, vitamin A may have an inhibitory effect on bladder carcinogens.

Several other cancers have been related to dietary factors. A high-animal-fat diet is a risk factor in cancer of the ovaries.[69] Iodine deficiency is a definite risk factor for thyroid cancer.[70]

Gastrointestinal cancers are the second leading cause of death among all cancer patients. Diet and nutrition are major risk factors in the development of gastrointestinal cancers and the others mentioned.[71] Smoking and alcohol consumption are also risk factors. All these risk factors *can be modified* by you: avoid beef and animal fat; eat low-cholesterol-containing foods; eat fiber-rich foods daily; eat green vegetables daily; stop smoking; drink alcohol in moderation; and do not take exogenous hormones (birth control pills, etc.). Finally, take the proper amount of vitamins and minerals as previously outlined as a food supplement. Antioxidants and vitamin A have been shown to be protective in colon cancers and other cancers.[72]

13

Cardiovascular Disease: Risk Factors in Common with Cancer

CARDIOVASCULAR disease is the leading cause of death in the United States. About 30 million Americans suffer from heart or blood vessel disease and as many as 27 million from high blood pressure. In 1978, 730,000 people died of heart disease and 190,000 died of stroke and other vascular complications—a total of 400 deaths per 100,000 people—and the death rate has increased since then. Cardiovascular disease accounts for 48 percent of all deaths in this country, compared to 22 percent caused by cancer. A quarter of the people who have a heart attack die within three hours of the first symptoms. Many don't even reach a hospital. Another 25 percent die within the first few weeks after a heart attack. Advances in intensive-care facilities throughout the United States probably will not significantly reduce the death rate from sudden death and can only partially affect patients in the hospital during the heart attack episode and convalescence. Furthermore, cardiovascular diseases cost the people and government of the United States over $52 billion a year; and more than $33 billion of this cost is related to premature death, or death before the age of 65. Once again we must learn about the risk factors involved and modify or eliminate them. We cannot cure the disease yet; we must try to prevent it. Nutrition has a great deal to do with heart disease, and many other risk factors for cancer are also risk factors for heart disease.

Most industrialized nations, except for Japan, have populations with a large incidence of heart disease. Japan, as we discussed in Chapter 12, has one of the lowest incidences of breast, colon, and prostate cancers in the world compared to other industrialized nations. A major risk factor for these cancers is nutrition: a high-animal-fat, high-cholesterol, low-fiber diet. Nutrition presents the same risk factor in heart disease: eating a low-animal-fat, low-cholesterol, high-fiber diet will decrease your risk of developing heart disease as well as breast, colon, and prostate cancers. It is known that atherosclerosis begins in childhood, so dietary modification and education should begin then also.

Atherosclerosis is responsible for the majority of all cardiovascular diseases (see pages 17–19). It is a disease which narrows the inside diameter of an artery. The first step in this narrowing is the manufacture of cells which line the inside of the artery. Then cholesterol gets deposited in these cells; this is called a plaque. Certain carcinogens can start the manufacture of these cells from a single cell. This process is called cloning, and it is a form of cancer. These carcinogens are hydrocarbons; they are carried in the blood by low-density lipoproteins (LDLs), which also carry cholesterol. LDLs are thought to be the initiators of the process of atherosclerosis. Therefore, if we eat food contaminated with hydrocarbons or

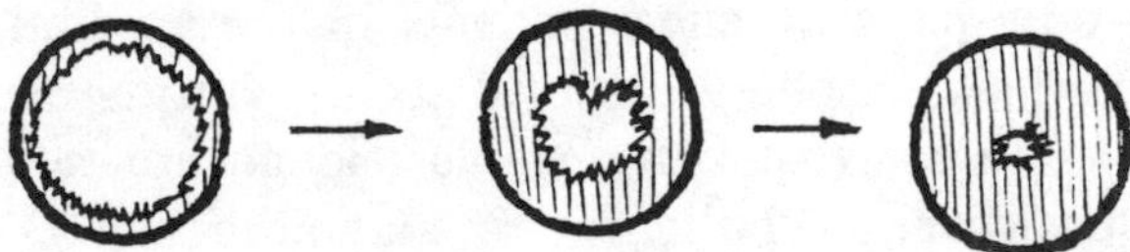

Figure 5. Progression of plaque formation

are otherwise exposed to them so that they can get into our bloodstream, atherosclerosis may begin. If the blood cholesterol is high, a plaque will form and begin to narrow the artery (see Figure 5).

These are the major risk factors for cardiovascular diseases:

1. High blood cholesterol
2. High blood lipids (triglycerides)
3. High blood pressure
4. Smoking
5. Age greater than 55
6. Obesity
7. Diabetes
8. Positive family history of *early* heart disease
9. Little or no physical activity.
10. Exogenous estrogens (birth control pills, etc.)
11. High-strung personality

Do any of these risk factors look familiar? Seven of the eleven cardiac risk factors are very important cancer risk factors as well.

Nutrition and Cardiovascular Disease

Dietary factors play a major role in determining the blood level of cholesterol and triglycerides. The Keys study was the first to show the correlation between heart disease and high cholesterol and lipids.[1] Since then eight or more international studies have confirmed this finding, including the recent Western Electric and Norwegian studies.[2,3] Another interesting study involved strict vegetarians who were asked to eat beef every day for two weeks. At the end of those two weeks their blood cholesterol had risen significantly, by 19 percent, and their blood pressure had risen slightly; both parameters returned to their normally low levels when they resumed their vegetarian diet.[4]

As dietary factors demonstrate pronounced differences for

cancer incidence in immigrant populations, so do dietary factors alter their cardiac disease rates. Japanese men living in Japan show a lower incidence of cardiovascular disease than Japanese-Americans in Hawaii or California, because of a lower blood cholesterol.

The Framingham study showed that the average intake of cholesterol was 650 mg per day for American men and 750 mg per day for American women.[5] Most of these people had cardiac disease.

Cholesterol is one of the three most important cardiac risk factors. Cholesterol is an important part of the atherosclerotic plaque. Animals fed high-cholesterol diets develop atherosclerosis. Regression of atherosclerosis in experimental animals is seen if they are fed a low-cholesterol diet. There are certain inherited forms of high blood cholesterol seen in a very few people; all these people have *early* heart disease. High blood lipids also contribute to heart disease. Eat low-animal-fat, low-cholesterol diets! I do not recommend lowering a high blood cholesterol level by eating more polyunsaturated fats. Polyunsaturated fats do have a lowering effect on the level of blood cholesterol, but, as we saw in Chapter 5, high levels of polyunsaturated fats in cell membranes can easily be attacked by free radicals and lead to the development of cancer.

In the past several years, there has been a lot of talk that low blood cholesterol is a risk factor for cancer. There is very little evidence to support this statement, however. It is true that one study showed a low blood cholesterol level in persons who also had cancer,[6] but four other studies showed no such correlation.[7] In fact, when information from six additional studies was reviewed, a low blood cholesterol level was associated with a very low risk of death from colon cancer.[8] There are more plausible reasons for the association of a low blood cholesterol level with cancer. First, the low blood cholesterol probably reflects the advanced degree of cancer rather than indicating a cause of cancer.[9] Second, people with colon cancer break down cholesterol, and these breakdown products are excreted out through the colon with the stool, so that the blood cholesterol level is low.[10]

Some foods may have a protective role in cardiovascular disease as well as in cancer. A fatty acid, eicosapentaenoic acid (EPA), which is found in most fish, especially salmon, and possibly in seaweed, lowers blood cholesterol and triglycerides and also reduces the tendency for blood clot formation. This finding has been confirmed[11,12,13,14] and suggests that fish should become a regular part of one's diet. Dietary fiber also plays a protective role in cardiovascular disease as well as in cancer. South African Bantu blacks were studied and found to have a much lower incidence of heart disease than white South Africans, probably because of their massive daily consumption of crude fiber.[15] As you will recall, these same Bantu peoples were studied by Oettle and were found to have a very low incidence of gastrointestinal cancer. Certain types of fiber, pectin, psyllium mucilloid, alfalfa, and guar gum cause decreases in blood cholesterol much more than do bran and other more crude fiber sources. Guar gum is derived from *Cyanopsis tragonolobus* and lowers the blood cholesterol level by an average of 13 percent, lowers the LDL level without altering the HDL level (high-density lipoproteins are believed to be protective), and lowers the blood glucose level.[16] Cholestyramine, a drug commonly used to treat patients with high blood cholesterol, was not tolerated as well as guar gum nor did it lower the blood cholesterol level to the same low degree as guar gum.[17] Psyllium mucilloid (Metamucil) and pectin (apples are best source) lower the cholesterol level but do not lower the LDL level. How fiber works is not clear, but many grains and fibers bind, or act as a glue for, bile acids. When the bile acids are bound, cholesterol cannot be absorbed from the gastrointestinal tract, because bile salts are needed for the transport of cholesterol from the gut to the blood. Therefore, dietary fiber should be eaten to decrease your risk of developing heart disease as well as cancer. Once again we see the benefit of a low-animal-fat, low-cholesterol, high-fiber diet.

High Blood Pressure

Hypertension, or high blood pressure, is another of the three major cardiac risk factors. It also is a risk factor for breast and colon cancer (see page 19). Blood pushes against your arteries as your heart beats. Sometimes this push is too great; then high blood pressure is the result. Hypertension is defined as having a blood pressure greater than 150/90. Two numbers make up the blood pressure. If either number or both are elevated consistently above those defined levels on more than three different office visits, a person then has hypertension by definition and should be treated on a daily basis. Hypertension represents an increased risk for developing stroke as well as heart disease. Of the people with hypertension, 95% have primary hypertension, the cause of which is unknown. The use of birth control pills is the second most common cause of high blood pressure.

High blood pressure increases with age and is 50 percent more likely to occur in American blacks than American whites. It affects over 35 million Americans and costs you and the government almost $15 billion per year. Adding salt (sodium chloride) to our food has been shown to increase the blood pressure by inducing a hormone called natriuretic to increase and thereby cause hypertension. Some studies are showing that adding salt to food may itself cause hypertension. In populations with low sodium intakes, hypertension is rare. Therefore, add minimal salt, if you must, to food while it is cooking. After the food is served, do not add more salt. Sodium is present in many beverages (soft drinks), processed foods, pickled foods, and sandwich meats. Americans consume about 2 teaspoons of salt per day, most of which is hidden in prepared foods, preservatives, and flavorings. Read the food labels. Limit your intake of salty foods such as potato chips, pretzels, nuts, cheese, pickled foods, and cured meat.

Smoking

Smoking is an extremely important risk factor for heart disease. Since the Surgeon General's report in 1964, there has been little doubt or controversy about the role of cigarette smoking in the development of heart attacks and cardiovascular disease. There is also little doubt concerning smoking as a risk factor for cancer.

Middle-aged adults have greatly reduced their cigarette smoking. But smoking among women as a whole and among teenagers has increased dramatically. The more a person smokes the more likely he or she is to have a heart attack. A person who smokes two packs of cigarettes a day is more at risk than someone who smokes one pack a day, and both are more likely to have a heart attack than a person who does not smoke at all. The likelihood of developing heart complications is greatly reduced when smoking is stopped. The Framingham study showed that heart disease is half as common among former smokers as among those who continue to smoke.[18] But more importantly, former smokers who haven't smoked for more than ten years seem to have the same risk as those who never smoked at all. (This does not apply to smokers who quit after the age of 65.) A person who smokes forty cigarettes a day has a risk of heart disease four times greater than a nonsmoker.

Smoking is a man-made cardiovascular and cancer risk factor, and thus can be modified. It you are presently smoking, it's up to you to stop! Smoking is one risk factor which will produce substantial results if modified.

Age

Age is another risk factor, but one that cannot be modified. We mentioned premature cardiac disease, which is inherited more often than not. However, the older you get past the age of 55, the greater your risk for cardiovascular disease if you have been eating the typical American diet all your life: high animal fat, high cholesterol, low fiber.

Obesity

Obesity together with one or more other risk factors seems to be a risk factor for cardiovascular disease. However, it appears from several studies that obesity by itself, without other concomitant factors like hypertension or diabetes, does not appear to be a major risk factor.[19,20]

Diabetes

Diabetes, another risk factor, is high blood sugar. About 80 percent of patients with both juvenile and adult onset diabetes die of some form of premature cardiovascular disease, usually heart attack. Diabetic men have twice as many cardiovascular problems as do nondiabetics, and diabetic women have three times as many. Diabetes is thought to adversely affect the blood vessel walls over the course of many years.

Family History

A person is at increased risk for heart disease if his mother, father, brother, or sister died of heart problems or heart attack before age 65. Of course, this is a risk factor that you can do very little about. You cannot pick and choose your parents. In addition to family history, males usually have a higher cardiac risk than females.

Physical Activity

It is widely thought that a less active person, especially in adult years, is more likely to have a heart attack. However, there is no firm evidence that exercise will increase life expectancy. Physical fitness does correlate with systolic blood pressure, lung capacity, and blood lipid levels (exercise raises the blood level of HDL, which is thought to be protective in heart disease[21]).

However, exercise itself can be dangerous. Anyone over the age of 35, or under the age of 35 with cardiac risk factors, should seek medical advice before beginning an exercise program.

Personality Factor

The role of stress is poorly understood in relation to cardiovascular disease. However, several studies show that an individual can be at risk for cardiac disease if he has a particular behavior or emotional life-style. This person is known as Type A personality, characterized by ambition, relentless drive, competitiveness, impatience, and being easily provoked. But these traits are difficult to quantitate, and hence studies of this type are difficult to interpret meaningfully.

Other Risk Factors

Oral hypoglycemic pills, which are medications other than insulin used to reduce blood sugar, seem to be a risk factor for cardiovascular disease, but this finding is very controversial. Women who use oral contraceptives have a three- to fourfold increased rate of heart attack, stroke, thrombophlebitis, and blood clots in the lung compared to women who never used them.[22] This risk is doubled in women who also smoke. Also there is a two- to threefold higher risk of having a heart attack even after a woman has stopped using oral contraceptives for five years or longer.[23]

Alcohol and caffeine have a possible role in cardiovascular disease. One large study done in 1977, the Cooperative Lipoprotein Phenotyping Study, which included 3806 people, has presented information that moderate consumption of alcohol may increase the HDL level (the cardiovascular protective lipoprotein).[24] The study shows that the HDL level increases modestly if a person consumes either a 12-ounce can of beer a day (0.60 ounces of 100 percent alcohol), a 4-ounce glass of wine a day (0.67 ounces of 100 percent alcohol), or a cocktail a day (0.69 ounces of 100 percent alcohol). Other studies have shown similar findings.[25,26,27] One additional study shows that persons who exercise vigorously every day, which alone will raise the HDL level, and consume a modest amount of alcohol daily will have a higher HDL level which is independent of the exercise factor.[28] Hence moderate amounts of alcohol alone will raise the HDL level whether a person exercises or not. These studies do not and cannot say that consuming this amount of these different drinks will decrease your risk of developing heart disease. It remains to be seen if such moderation in alcohol consumption will have any positive impact on heart disease. Excessive alcohol consumption is very harmful. It can directly produce an irreversibly enlarged heart and is related to several different cancers as well and many other complications of alcoholism. Caffeine can stimulate the heart to beat faster, which is harmful for a person who has coronary artery disease.

Many of these risk factors can be and should be modified; it will lessen your risk of developing cardiovascular disease. Recently, ABC News commentators interviewed doctors at the Arizona Heart Institute on *60 Minutes* concerning the institute's "Cardiovascular Risk Factor Analysis." This consists of a list of risk factors, each followed by statements of which you choose one, and a score associated with the statement. After going through the questionnaire, add up your numerical score.

Risk Factor	Statement	Score	
1. Age	Over 55 years of age	Score 1	
	Under 55 years of age	Score 0	______
2. Gender	Male	Score 1	
	Female	Score 0	______
3. Family History	If one or more close family member had heart attack before age of 60	Score 12	

Risk Factor	Statement	Score	
	If one or more had heart attack after age 60	Score 6	
	No family history	Score 0	______
4. Personal History	If you had heart attack, stroke or heart or blood vessel surgery before age 50	Score 20	
	If you had the above after age 50	Score 10	
	If you had none	Score 0	______
5. Diabetes	Onset before age 40 using insulin	Score 10	
	Onset after 40 using insulin or pills	Score 5	
	No diabetes or diet controlled	Score 0	______
6. Smoking	Smoke 2 packs or more per day	Score 10	
	Smoke 1–2 packs or quit less than a year ago	Score 6	
	Smoke less than 1 pack or quit 1–10 years ago	Score 3	
	Never smoked or quit 10 years ago	Score 0	______
7. Cholesterol	If blood level over 275	Score 10	
	If level between 225 and 275	Score 5	
	If level below 225	Score 0	______
8. Diet	One serving of red meat daily, 7 eggs a week, and use butter, milk, and cheese daily	Score 8	

Risk Factor	Statement	Score	
	Red meat 5–6 times a week, 4–7 eggs a week, margarine, low-fat dairy products and some cheese	Score 4	
	Little or no red meat, but rather poultry and fish, 3 eggs or less, margarine, skim milk, and skim milk products	Score 0	_______
9. Hypertension	If pressure is above 160 over 105	Score 8	
	Between 140 to 160 over 90 to 105	Score 4	
	Lower than 140 over 90	Score 0	_______
10. Weight	Ideal weight for men should be 110 pounds plus 5 lbs per inch over 5 ft. For women, ideal weight is 100 lbs plus 5 lbs per inch over 5 ft		
	If you are 25 lbs overweight	Score 4	
	If you are 10–25 lbs over	Score 2	
	If you are less than 10 lbs over	Score 0	_______
11. Exercise	If you briskly walk, jog, bicycle, swim, etc. for 15 minutes only once a week	Score 4	

Risk Factor	Statement	Score	
	Those exercises twice a week	Score 2	
	Those exercises 3 or more times a week	Score 0	______
12. Stress	If you are frustrated waiting in line, easily angered or irritable	Score 4	
	Occasionally harried or moody	Score 2	
	Comfortable when waiting, easygoing	Score 0	______
		TOTAL POINTS	______

The Arizona Heart Institute defines risk for having cardiovascular disease based on the following total point score:

High Risk	Score of 40 or over
Medium Risk	Score of 20 to 39
Low Risk	Score of 19 or under

A high score does not mean a person will develop heart disease; the test only indicates that a person with a high score is more at risk than a person with a low score.

FOUR

Modifying the Risks

14

Exercise and Relaxation

EXERCISE, CANCER, AND CARDIAC FITNESS

ABOUT 25 million Americans jog regularly because they have heard the popular notion that strenuous exercise will protect them from coronary heart disease. There have been several extreme claims concerning the beneficial effects of exercise. T. J. Bassler says that if a person has the conditioning to finish in a 26-mile marathon, he will not develop heart disease. However, a marathon runner did have a cardiac arrest and died while running, a victim of coronary heart disease. But there is good evidence now that physical inactivity is a risk factor for cardiovascular disease.

Exercise may be beneficial by positively influencing other risk factors such as cholesterol and high blood pressure. Exercise raises the level of high-density-lipoprotein cholesterol, which exerts a protective effect in coronary heart disease.[1] Exercise may reduce a moderately high blood pressure to normal in an obese person who has lost weight by exercising. Also, if an obese person is diabetic and requires insulin to regulate his sugar, then exercise will decrease that person's weight and thereby decrease insulin requirements. A person with a Type A personality (competitive, impatient, irritable, etc.) may also benefit from exercising because of some physical improvements as well as psychological changes, which include feeling relaxed and having less severe mood swings. There is one study which shows angiographically (dye injected into coronary arteries) that coronary artery disease will slow down with regular exercise.[2] This finding has not been confirmed, however.

There have been several animal studies that show that exercise inhibits tumor growth.[3,4] However, two human studies show that people who do not exercise much do not have a higher incidence of cancer than those who exercise a fair amount.[5,6] Presently, from the information available in the scientific literature, it cannot be concluded that exercise will influence cancer development or growth.

The main risk of beginning an exercise program is sudden death. Most reported cases of sudden death are older persons who had several cardiac risk factors. Among the non-life-threatening adverse effects of jogging and running are those ranging from blister formation to bursitis, Achilles tendonitis to stress fracture, and possibly early osteoarthritis, a wearing out of bones. Long-distance runners can transiently have blood in their urine. Other problems associated with jogging include heat stroke and problems related to breast connective tissue support.

Because of a risk of sudden death associated with beginning to exercise, anyone 35 years or older, or under 35 with cardiac risk factors, should be medically screened. This screening should include a full history and physical examination by a physician, and a resting electrocardiogram (ECG). An exercise electrocardiogram is indicated if the person has symptoms of heart disease.

An exercise program should be individualized for each person because abilities and motivations differ. Activities that offer a constant and sustained exertion (like fast walking, running, and swimming) may offer physiological advantages over activities with varying levels of exertion (like volleyball and tennis).

The exercise program should start slowly and then gradually build up to the desired level. The heart rate should be monitored. The safest training program is one in which training lasts twenty to forty minutes per day, three to four times a week, while maintaining the heart rate during exercise at 50 percent of the predicted maximum heart rate for the age of the person.[7] Of course, the person should be warned to stop exercising immediately if he experiences chest pain, severe shortness of breath, palpitations, or other cardiac symptoms. He should contact his physician at once.

About how many people are engaged in an exercise program? The Perrier survey interviewed 1510 adults at random and found that 59 percent of them were actively exercising in one form or another, but only 15 percent spent more than five hours per week exercising—equivalent to about 1500 calories per week. Running was ranked sixth in popularity behind walking, swimming, calisthenics, bicycling, and bowling. Not all would be likely to improve cardiovascular fitness. Only about 5 percent of the adults were doing meaningful exercises which would actually improve cardiac fitness. The survey concluded the one most important factor likely to initiate and increase a person's physical activity was his physician's recommendation.[8]

Nutrition and Exercise

The new athlete often consults with his physician about matters which are related to exercise and nutrition. Young and old athletes alike realize that proper nutrition plays a big role in their performance. Over 7 million high-school athletes are in an age group which has the highest risk of nutritional deficiencies.[9] An adequate diet, with the proper vitamin and mineral supplementation if necessary, is a must for all athletes. Athletes who are their ideal weight may require additional calories for the extra energy they need. They can monitor this by weighing themselves regularly to see if their daily dietary intake meets the needs of routine activities plus training requirements. Do not increase muscle mass by taking any hormones like testosterone (which is a risk factor for cancer). Exercising your muscles will increase your muscle mass.

RELAXATION

It is very important for a person to relax and deal with stress in a controlled manner, especially for those who have a Type A personality. An experiment was set up to see what effect stress had on the rejection of cancer. Three groups of rats were given cancer. One group received electric shock treatments but was allowed to escape from it if it wanted; the second group received the same electric shock, but for these rats there was no escape route; and the third group did not receive any electric shocks. About 63 percent of the rats receiving escapable shock and 54 percent of the rats receiving no shock rejected the cancer, but only 27 percent of the rats receiving inescapable shock rejected the cancer.[10] These results imply that if an animal is able to control stress, then that animal can also reject cancer much better than an animal which cannot control stress.

Relaxation should be individualized; what may be relaxing for you may actually annoy and create anxiety for another. Relaxation is usually not accomplished in a noisy setting, however. Obviously, if young children are running about the house and the television is blaring, it is more difficult to relax.

Get into a very comfortable lounging position. Concentrate on "feeling" with your mind every part of your body. You can begin by thinking about your right foot, then your right ankle, right leg, right thigh, then left foot, etc.; then from your hands up to your shoulders and neck, and so on. Now start to tense specific muscle groups as hard as you can, hold them tense for twenty to thirty seconds, then relax them. Again, start with your foot muscles (tense, relax), the leg muscles (tense, relax), and so on. You can repeat the entire sequence once or twice. While you are doing this, tell yourself that you are tightening your muscles each time you do so, and, provided that your effort is exhausting, you will look forward to relaxing each muscle group. While this is happening, you can also think of a pleasant place that invokes fond memories. This sequence should produce relief and relaxation and decrease your anxiety levels.

15

Ten-Point Plan for Risk Factor Modification

CANCER, the most dread of all diseases, will affect one out of every three to four Americans. Eighty to 90 percent of all cancers are related to nutritional factors (a high-animal-fat, high-cholesterol, low-fiber diet), life-style (tobacco smoking, excessive alcohol consumption), the environment (chemical carcinogens, ozone, air pollution, industrial exposure), and some hormones and drugs. As we have learned, many of these cancer risk factors are risk factors for developing and worsening cardiovascular diseases as well. Since we can now identify many of these factors, we should modify them accordingly to lessen our risk of developing cancer and cardiovascular diseases. The likelihood of drastically increasing the number of cancer cures by conventional cancer therapies in the foreseeable future is not great, even though some of the very best American minds and technologies are involved in cancer research.

Cancer is the most complex group of diseases known, and there are many different causes. We must all do our part to try to *prevent* cancer, because that is how the number of new cancer cases can be substantially reduced. Americans need to know the risk factors for cancer and cardiovascular diseases. Adults who learn these risk factors and then modify their diet and life-style accordingly will reduce their risk for developing cancer and cardiovascular diseases. Children will benefit the most from properly modified nutritional factors and daily habits. Nutrition education should be part of a child's education throughout the school years, because nutritional practices and habits are easily modified in youth. Nutrition is a topic of extreme interest to teachers and parents as well. The main risk factors for the development of cancer and cardiovascular disease are nutrition and tobacco smoking. If parents set the example of correct nutritional practices, no smoking, and very modest alcohol consumption, their children will continue these practices throughout their own lives. There will be a consequent decrease in the incidence of cancer and cardiovascular disease.

What can you do to help yourself? My recommendations to modify your risk factors for cancer as well as cardiovascular disease will not be anything like the popular fad diets or the crash schemes for weight reduction, longevity, or reversal of cardiovascular or other diseases.[1] Primary prevention and early detection are the goals of my plan for risk factor modification—no fads, no claims for disease-free longevity. Simply, I have presented the current body of scientific information concerning cancer and cardiovascular disease risk factors, and now will discuss how those risk factors can be modified. The more closely you adhere to my recommendations, the better off you will be.

POINT 1: NUTRITION

While it is reasonable to conclude that high dietary animal fat, cholesterol, low fiber intake, obesity, and possibly other nutrients may be responsible for certain cancers and heart disease, the data are not 100 percent conclusive. However, the preponderance of information suggests the following.

Maintain an ideal weight. You will find several medically sound weight reduction diets in the next chapter, along with a table of foods and their compositions.

Consume a low-animal-fat, low-cholesterol diet. Eating the recommended foods under this heading will provide you with more than enough fats necessary for all bodily functions and at the same time modify disease risks.

1. *Eat poultry.* White meat is best. Remove all skin before cooking. Chicken, turkey, Cornish hen, and game birds are good. Do not eat any fatty poultry like goose or duck.
2. *Eat fish.* All fish is recommended except scallops, shellfish, sardines, mackerel, other fatty fish, and fish canned in oil. These exceptions are high in fat or cholesterol.
3. *Limit red meat.* Eat only lean red meat and limit consumption to about once a week. Eliminate all fatty meats like bacon, fatty hamburger, spareribs, sausage, lunch meats, sweetbreads, hot dogs, kidney, brains, liver, etc. Do not smoke, charcoal broil, barbecue or salt-cure foods.
4. *Eat soybeans and soybean products.*
5. *Limit dairy products.* Only nonfat products (up to 1 percent by weight) should be eaten: skim milk, skim powdered milk, evaporated skim milk, nonfat yogurt and buttermilk, and only cheeses made with skim milk or 1 percent fat milk. Eat only a few egg whites per week or cholesterol-free egg substitute a couple of times a week. Eliminate whole milk and low-fat milk and products made from them, cream, half and half, all cheeses containing greater than 1 percent fat, whipped cream, etc. Do not eat whole eggs.
6. *Eliminate all oils and fats* including butter, margarine, meat fat, lard, and all oils. Both saturated and polyunsaturated fats are detrimental.
7. *Watch garnishes and sauces.* Use products which do not have fats, oils, or egg yolks. Dry white wine may be used in cooking, and you can also use ketchup and vinegar. Do not

use salad dressings, pickle relish, prepared gravies and sauces, mayonnaise, sandwich spreads, or other products containing fats, oils, or egg yolks.

Eat a high-fiber-content diet. Consume foods which will give you 12 to 15 grams of fiber content per day. Consult Chapter 16 for the fiber content of foods. As you will learn, it is very easy to choose foods which will give you a total of 15 grams of fiber a day.

Vegetables of the Brassicaceae family, as well as providing fiber, can induce enzymes to destroy certain carcinogens. These include brussels sprouts, broccoli, and cabbage. You can eat all whole or lightly milled grains like rice, barley, and buckwheat. Whole wheat bread and whole wheat pasta, cereals, crackers, and other grain products can also be eaten. Unsweetened fruit juices and unsweetened cooked, canned, or frozen fruit can also be eaten.

Do not eat cooked, canned, or frozen fruit with added sugar, all jams and jellies, fruit syrups with added sugars, fruit juices with added sugars, bleached white flour, and grain products made with added fats, oils, or egg yolks. Avoid butter rolls, commercial biscuits, muffins, donuts, sweet rolls, cakes, egg bread, cheese bread, and commercial mixes containing dried eggs and whole milk.

Vitamins and minerals. You should supplement your balanced diet with vitamins and minerals in the proper dosages and combinations so that risks are even further modified. The formulation I have developed, the "Risk Modifier™," is outlined in Chapter 6. It contains effective doses of all the vitamins and selected minerals, especially antioxidants. General Nutrition Corporation has manufactured the "Risk Modifier™" to my specifications and will have it in convenient tablet form. However, you may wish to obtain individual vitamins and minerals in these doses.

Salt. Eliminate table salt. Add only a minimal amount of salt while cooking. Most condiments, pickles, dressings, prepared sauces, canned vegetables, bouillon cubes, pot pies, popcorn, sauerkraut, and caviar have high amounts of salt in them.

Food additives. Avoid all foods containing nitrates, nitrites, and other harmful additives and processing techniques.

Snacks and desserts. Acceptable snacks or desserts include fresh fruit and canned fruit without added sugar, water ices, gelatin, and (sparingly) puddings made with skim milk. Do not eat commercial cakes, pies, cookies, donuts, and mixes; coconut or coconut oil; frozen cream pies; potato chips and other deep-fried snacks; whole milk puddings; ice cream; candy; chocolate; or gum with sugar.

Beverages. Acceptable beverages are skim milk or nonfat buttermilk, mineral water, unsweetened fruit juices, and vegetable juices. Consume in moderation caffeine-containing beverages—coffee, tea, colas, etc.—and avoid chemically decaffeinated drinks.

Dining out. Call the restaurant to see if they can accommodate your needs as outlined here. Airlines and ocean liners will also help you. Request that the chef not cook with any salt products (Chinese food is high in sodium). Use lemon juice or vinegar on your salad.

POINT 2: TOBACCO

Do not smoke! Do not chew tobacco. If you are smoking, quit now. There is no easy, painless way to quit. The best way is simply to go "cold turkey" without tapering off or using any of those expensive smoke-ending courses (see Chapter 9). The American Lung Association can help you. Call them. Remember, cigarette smoke also endangers the health of nonsmokers.

POINT 3: ALCOHOL

Alcoholic beverages may be consumed in moderation: 4 ounces of wine per day, 12 ounces of beer per day, or one mixed drink per day. Alcoholic beverages in these amounts increase the HDL level, which is useful only if the blood cholesterol level is high.

POINT 4: RADIATION

X-ray exposure (ionizing). X-ray pictures are certainly needed in many circumstances and should be taken when a physician recommends it. The equipment is getting better and less rad is delivered to a person per film now. However, there are hypochondriacs who want X-ray studies, and some people involved in motor vehicle accidents also want X-rays done for possible legal purposes. These people receive unnecessary radiation exposure.

See a physician if you had radiation to your head and neck as a child.

Sunlight. Sun screens should be used when you sunbathe. Remember, sunlight causes skin cancer and ages skin rapidly. Avoid suntanning booths.

POINT 5: ENVIRONMENTAL EXPOSURE

Environmental protection standards for air, water, and the work place should be rigorously observed.

Several specific industries, such as the manufacturing of boots, shoes, furniture, and cabinets, are risk factors for developing cancer of the nasal sinuses. Other industries which use certain chemicals (see Chapter 2, Table II) pose an increased risk for persons working with those chemicals. All these industries have safety standards which should be strictly observed. For instance, a person working with asbestos (insulation, brake lining, etc.) should wear a mask to protect the respiratory and gastrointestinal systems. Frequently workers find a mask to be a nuisance and will not wear one, especially on hot days. This simply increases their risk for developing cancer. Firefighters are indirectly exposed to many of these chemicals when objects made from them burn. A study should investigate how much higher, if at all, the incidence of several cancers is among firefighters.

Avoid prolonged exposure to household cleaning fluids, solvents, and paint thinners. Some may be hazardous if inhaled in high concentrations. Pesticides, fungicides, and other home garden and lawn chemicals are also potentially dangerous. When you handle them follow the label instructions, wash your hands afterward, and store the chemicals in a place where children cannot get at them.

POINT 6: SEXUAL-SOCIAL FACTORS, HORMONES, AND DRUGS

Female promiscuity. The earlier the age of starting sexual intercourse and the more male sexual partners a female has (particularly uncircumcised partners), the higher is her risk of developing cancer of the cervix.

Hygiene in uncircumcised males. Bathe frequently. Poor hygiene may lead to cancer of the penis.

Male homosexuality (promiscuity and/or amyl nitrite use). The immune system of many sexually active male homosexuals is severely impaired if they have many male partners and/or if they use amyl nitrite. Both of these situations are risk factors for Kaposi's sarcoma. The sexually active male homosexual also is at risk for developing cancer of the anus and cancer of the tongue.

Birth control pills. Birth control pills should not be used, nor should estrogens be used to treat other conditions. Other means of birth control should be sought.

DES exposure. Report to a physician if you yourself were exposed to DES, or if you are the daughter or son of a DES-exposed mother.

Androgens. Androgens (those substituted with a methyl compound in the seventeenth position) should not be used for body building or any other purpose. Build your body by working out.

Drugs. Avoid all unnecessary drugs. Take drugs only when they are prescribed by your physician. Check to see if the drug interferes with vitamin function.

POINT 7: LEARN THE SEVEN CANCER WARNING SIGNS

Lump or thickening of breast

A change in a wart or a mole

A sore that does not heal

Change in bowel or bladder habits

Persistent cough or hoarseness

Constant indigestion or trouble swallowing

Unusual bleeding or discharge

If any of these signs appear, contact your physician immediately.

POINT 8: CANCER QUESTIONNAIRE*

(If after answering these questions, you find you have three or more or all of the possible yes answers in any one category, consult your physician.)

General	No	Yes
1. Have you ever been told by a physician that you had cancer?	___	___
If yes, cancer of what? ______		
2. Have any of your blood relatives had cancer?	___	___
If yes, cancer of what? ______		
3. Have you lost 10 to 15 pounds over the past 6 months without knowing why?	___	___
Lungs		
4. Have you coughed up blood in the past several weeks?	___	___
5. Have you had a chronic daily cough?	___	___
6. Have you been told that you have emphysema?	___	___
7. Have you had pneumonia twice or more in the past year?	___	___
8. Have you ever smoked?	___	___
9. Did you quit smoking 15 years ago or more?	___	___

* Adopted from Cancer Prevention and Detection Screening Program.

Lungs			No	Yes
10. Do you smoke now?			___	___
Cigarettes:	Number of packs/day	___ .		
	Number of years	___ .		
Cigars:	Number of cigars/day	___ .		
Pipe:	Number of bowls/day	___ .		

Larynx (voice box)		
11. Have you had persistent hoarseness?	___	___
Mouth and Throat		
12. Have you had any of the following symptoms lasting more than a month?	___	___
Pain or difficulty swallowing	___	___
Pain or tenderness in the mouth	___	___
A sore or white spot in your mouth	___	___
13. Do you drink more than 4 oz. of wine, 12 oz. of beer, or 1½ oz. of whiskey every day?	___	___
Stomach		
14. Have you vomited blood in the past month?	___	___
15. Have you had black stools in the past 6 months?	___	___
Does this happen only when you are taking pills with iron in them?	___	___
16. Have you had a stomach pain several times a week?	___	___
17. Has a physician told you that you had stomach growths called polyps or an ulcer?	___	
Large Intestine and Rectum		
18. Have you had a change in your usual bowel habits?	___	___
19. Has your stool been becoming more narrow in diameter?	___	___
20. Does this happen with every bowel movement?	___	___

Large Intestine and Rectum	No	Yes
21. Have you had bleeding from the rectum, either with bowel movements or at other times?	___	___
22. Have you had mucus in your stool every time you had a bowel movement?	___	___
23. Have you been told that you had a polyp in the large intestine?	___	___
24. Have you had ulcerative colitis?	___	___

Breasts

	No	Yes
25. Do you self-examine your breasts?	___	___
26. Do you have a lump in either breast?	___	___
27. Have you had breast pain recently?	___	___
If yes, is this only at time of menstruation?	___	___
28. Has there been discharge or bleeding from your nipples, or have they begun to pull in (retract)?	___	___
29. Are there any changes in the skin of your breasts?	___	___
30. Have you ever had a breast biopsy?	___	___

Cervix, Uterus, and Vagina

	No	Yes
31. Do you have vaginal bleeding or spotting?	___	___
If yes:		
Is it between periods?	___	___
Is it after sexual intercourse?	___	___
Is it after menopause?	___	___
32. Have you stopped having your periods?	___	___
At what age? ______		
Since then, have you ever had hormone therapy?	___	___
Have you had a hysterectomy?	___	___
33. Have you ever had sexual intercourse?	___	___
Did you first have intercourse before age 16?	___	___

Cervix, Uterus, and Vagina	No	Yes
34. Did your mother use the hormone DES when she was pregnant with you?	__	__
Skin		
35. Has there been bleeding or a change in a mole on your body?	__	__
36. Do you have a mole on your body where it may be irritated by underwear, a belt, etc.?	__	__
37. Do you have a sore that does not heal?	__	__
38. Do you have a severe scar from a burn?	__	__
39. Do you have fair skin and sunburn easily?	__	__
40. Do you sunbathe for long hours or use a suntanning booth?	__	__
Thyroid		
41. Can you see or feel a lump in the lower front of your neck?	__	__
42. Did you have X-ray treatment to your face for acne, tonsil enlargement, or other reasons?	__	__
Kidney and Urinary Bladder		
43. Have you had blood in your urine?	__	__

POINT 9: EXERCISE

Everyone should start a program of exercise, but see a physician before doing so if you have risk factors of cardiovascular disease (see Chapter 13). Initially the exercising should start out slowly, then increase to a comfortable level. Fast walking is a good form of exercise and should be done as part of your program. Two miles would be a satisfactory distance to fast walk four out of seven days. I stress fast walking because it is easier to do than other forms of exercise—no equipment to buy, no change of clothing, no one else to rely on except yourself. You can walk in a shopping mall in inclement weather. Calisthenics should also be done to firm up abdominal wall muscles and decrease that "spare tire." Five to ten sit-ups, with knees bent, can readily be done at home every day. Remember, some exercise is better than none. Choose exercises that you will adhere to and continue as part of your life-style modification.

POINT 10: EXECUTIVE PHYSICAL

It is well known that persons with localized cancer are potentially curable and live longer than those with widespread cancer. Hence everyone age 35 and older should have an annual comprehensive executive-type history and physical examination with appropriate laboratory studies, in order to prevent or detect early cancer or heart disease. What is certain is that if a physician looks for early cancer, he will probably find it if it is there.

A thorough history should include questions about all the risk factors for cancer which are listed in Chapter 2, as well as a review of the questions outlined in Point 8 above. Also, questions should be asked concerning the risk factors of cardiovascular disease (see Chapter 13) as well as other routine questions which are designed to pick up additional medical abnormalities.

The physical examination is important and should be complete, starting at the scalp and finishing at the toes. One capable, highly trained specialist should perform the entire examination, rather than your gynecologist doing the Pap smear and breast exam, your cardiologist checking the heart, your dentist looking in your mouth, and so on. The examining physician can then ask for consultation in certain circumstances. Indirect laryngoscopy (a look at the vocal cords), toluidine blue dye mouth rinse, and sigmoidoscopy should also be done in high-risk patients.

Laboratory tests are the third major part of a person's workup. Little more than one ounce of blood and urine is taken and assayed for chemical tests. Table I lists the laboratory tests, the normal range values of the tests, and the functions tested.

Testing the stool for trace amounts of blood is another important laboratory examination. Trace amounts of blood in the stool have their origins from some lesion(s) in the gastrointestinal tract, which could be a gastrointestinal cancer. To detect the reason for the blood, the gastrointestine should then be appropriately worked up by doing a sigmoidoscopy, air-contrast barium enema, etc. It is important to completely avoid all red meat for three entire days prior to and during the collection of the stool specimens, because red meat contains animal blood, which will produce a positive result in the test.

A chest X-ray and resting electrocardiogram should be a standard part of a workup to assess a person's heart and lungs—two very vital organs. If the resting electrocardiogram is abnormal or if a person has cardiac symptoms, an exercise or stress electrocardiogram should be done by a competent specialist. A person's lung function can be readily assessed by spirometry, a test which determines the quantity and speed of the air moving in and out, the volumes of the lungs, etc. In addition, L. B. Woolner and colleagues have reported that routine examination of sputum specimens (excretions brought up from the lungs) in specific high-risk patients will detect certain cancers earlier.[2]

If a bruit (pronounced brew-ee) is heard in a person's neck and the person has no strokelike symptoms from this abnormality, special tests should be done to determine if the all-impor-

Table I

Laboratory Test	Normal Range	Function Tested
Cholesterol	160–260	Blood lipids
HDL-cholesterol	25–90	
Triglycerides	10–150	
Alkaline phosphatase	30–85	Liver function and enzymes
SGPT	3–44	
SGOT	8–31	
LDH	133–248	
Total bilirubin	.2–1.5	
Total protein	6.1–7.7	Blood proteins
Albumin	3.8–4.9	
Blood urea nitrogen	7–23	Kidney function
Creatinine	.7–1.6	
Urinalysis		
Glucose	70–120	Blood sugar
Calcium	4.5–5.3	Electrical function of cells
Phosphate	3.0–4.5	
Magnesium	1.3–2.1	
Sodium	137–145	
Chloride	100–110	
Potassium	3.3–4.6	
CO_2	23–33	
Uric acid	3–7	
Hemoglobin	Male: 13–16; Female: 12–15	Blood count
Hematocrit	Male: 42–50; Female: 40–48	
White blood cells	5,000–10,000	
Platelet count	145,000–365,000	
Stool for occult blood	Negative	Bleeding from gut

tant carotid arteries are severely narrowed. A bruit is a sound heard in an artery, usually produced by obstructions caused by plaques in the arteries.

A breast examination also should routinely be performed in the intervening time between executive physicals.

Table II shows which cancer(s) can be detected in each part of the executive examination.

Table II

CANCER DETECTED BY EACH PART OF EXECUTIVE EXAMINATION

Part of Executive Examination	Cancer Detected
Medical history	Most cancers with local or generalized symptoms
Executive physical examination	Skin, lymphoma, mouth, thyroid, breast, abdominal, uterus, vagina, rectum, penis, testicle
Chest X-ray	Lung, pleura, central chest, bone
Complete blood count	Leukemias, multiple myeloma, cancers that produce abnormal red and white counts
Blood chemistries	Liver and associated cancer, kidney
Urinalysis	Kidney, bladder
Stool occult blood	Gastrointestine
Papanicolaou smear	Uterine cervix
Sputum cytology	Lung
Mammography	Breast
Sigmoidoscopy	Rectum and sigmoid colon
Indirect laryngoscopy	Larynx
Toluidine blue mouth rinse	Mouth

CANCER RISK FACTOR ASSESSMENT

My Cancer Risk Factor Assessment Test follows. Take the test. After you begin to modify your risk factors according to my recommendations, take the test again to see if your overall risk has been reduced.

The test consists of a list of cancer risk factors, several statements associated with each risk factor, and a specified score associated with each statement. Choose the statement that most nearly applies to you and write its score in the blank. After going through the questionnaire, add up your scores. The zero scores won't count in the total.

CANCER RISK FACTOR ASSESSMENT

Risk Factor	Statement	Score
1. *Nutrition*	If during 50% or more of your life 2 or more of the following apply to you: (1) one serving of red meat daily (including lunch meat); (2) 6 eggs per week; (3) use butter, milk, or cheese daily; (4) little or no fiber foods (3 gm or less) daily; (5) frequent barbecued meats; (6) below-average intake of vitamins and minerals.	Score A ____
	If during 50% or more of your life 2 or more of the following apply to you: (1) red meat 4–5 times per week (including lunch meat); (2) 3–5 eggs per week; (3) margarine, low-fat dairy products, some cheese; (4) 4–7 gm of fiber daily; (5) average intake of vitamins and minerals.	Score B ____

Risk Factor	Statement	Score
	If during 50% or more of your life 2 or more of the following apply to you:	
	(1) red meat and 1 egg once a week or none at all;	
	(2) poultry or fish daily or very frequently;	
	(3) margarine, skim milk, and skim milk products;	
	(4) 12–15 gm of fiber daily;	
	(5) above-average intake of vitamins and minerals.	Score 0 _____
2. *Weight*	Ideal weight for men is 110 lbs plus 5 lbs per inch over 5 ft. For women, ideal weight is 100 lbs plus 5 lbs per inch over 5 ft.	
	If you are 25 lbs overweight.	Score B
	If you are 10–24 lbs over.	Score C
	If you are less than 10 lbs over.	Score 0 _____
3. *Tobacco*	Smoke 2 packs or more per day for 10 years or more.	Score A
	Smoke 1–2 packs for 10 years or more or quit less than a year ago.	Score A
	Smoke less than 1 pack for 10 years or more or smoke pipe or cigar.	Score B

	Smoked 1–2 packs per day or pipe or cigar but stopped 7–14 years ago.	Score B	
	Chew or snuff tobacco.	Score B	
	Never smoked or quit 15 years ago.	Score 0	_____
4. *Occupation*	If you are a radiologist, chemist, painter, uranium or hematite miner, luminous-dial painter, or a worker in the following industries: leather, foundry, printing, rubber, petroleum, furniture or cabinet, textile, nuclear, slaughterhouse, or plutonium. (The longer your exposure, the greater your risk.)	Score B	
	Never was one of the above workers.	Score 0	_____
5. *Chemicals*	If you have worked directly with one of the following chemicals: aniline, acrylonitrile, 4-aminobiphenyl, arsenic, asbestos, auramine manufacturing, benzene, benzidene, beryllium, cadmium, carbon tetrachloride, chlormethyl ether, chloroprene, chromate, isopropyl alcohol (acid process), nickel, mustard gas, or vinyl chloride. (The longer your exposure, the higher your risk.)	Score A	
	If you have worked indirectly with one of the above chemicals.	Score C	
	Never worked with one of the above.	Score 0	_____

Risk Factor	Statement	Score
6. *Immunity, drugs, and hormones*	If your physician said you have a severe deficiency in your immune system, or you have received an organ transplant.	Score A
	If you have taken one or more of the following for a prolonged period of time: chlorambucil, cyclophosphamide, melphalan, or high-dose steroids (anticancer drugs).	Score A
	If you have taken one or more of the following for a prolonged period of time: phenacetin, thiotepa, diethylstilbestrol (DES), birth control pills (conjugated estrogens), or 17 methyl-substituted androgens.	
	If you had early onset of menses or late onset of menopause, or never had menses at all.	Score B
	If you were first pregnant late in life or never at all, or had fibrocystic breast disease.	Score C
	If none of the above apply.	Score 0 ____
7. *Alcohol*	If you drink 4 oz or more of whiskey daily or equivalent alcohol content in other beverages.	Score B
	If you drink the same quantity as above and also smoke:	
	Less than 1 pack per day or chew or snuff tobacco.	Score B
	1–2 packs per day, pipe, or cigar.	Score A
	2 or more packs per day.	Score A
	Moderate or social drinking, or no drinking at all.	Score 0 ____

8. *Occult cancer signs and symptoms*	If you have one or more of the 7 Cancer Warning Signs or have answered yes to 4 or more of the abnormal signs and symptoms in the Cancer Questionnaire.	Score B	
	If you have one of the 7 Cancer Warning signs and have answered yes to less than 4 of the abnormal signs and symptoms in the Cancer Questionnaire.	Score C	
	If you have none or answered no.	Score 0	_____
9. *Geography*	Based on Figure 1 in Chapter 1, if during most of your life you lived in one of the states with the most cancer deaths.	Score B	
	If during most of your life you lived in a state that has a moderate number of cancer deaths.	Score C	
	If during most of your life you lived in a state with the least number of cancer deaths.	Score 0	_____
10. *Age*	If your age is 70 or more.	Score B	
	If your age is 55 to 69.	Score C	
	If your age is 55 or under.	Score 0	_____
11. *Personal history*	If you had cancer.	Score B	
	If you never had cancer.	Score 0	_____
12. *Family history*	If one or more close family members had cancer.	Score B	
	No family history of cancer.	Score 0	_____

Risk Factor	Statement	Score
13. *Sexual-social history*	If you are a female who started having sexual intercourse before age 16 and has had many male partners, particularly uncircumcised.	Score C
	If you are a sexually active male homosexual who has had many male partners and/or uses amyl nitrite.	Score C
	If neither applies.	Score 0 ____
14. *Radiation exposure*	If you received multiple X-rays, radiation treatments, or were exposed to: radioactive isotopes used for diagnostic workups, or atomic or thermonuclear weapons.	Score C
	If you are fair-skinned and sunburn easily.	Score B
	If neither applies.	Score 0 ____
15. *Stress*	If you are frustrated waiting in line, easily angered, and unable to control stress.	Score C
	If you are comfortable when waiting, easygoing, and able to control stress.	Score 0 ____

TOTAL SCORE: ____ A's; ____ B's; and ____ C's.

We define risk for potentially developing cancer based on the following letter combination totals:

High risk	2 or more A's + any number of B's or C's or 1 A + 4 or more B's + any number of C's
Moderate risk	1 A + 3 or fewer B's + any number of C's or 4 or more B's + any number of C's or 2 or 3 B's + 2 or more C's
Low risk	No A's or No B's or no C's or 1 B + 2 or fewer C's or 2 or fewer C's

A person in a high-risk category will not necessarily develop cancer. The high-risk category indicates only that a person in it is more at risk than a person in another category.

Here are a few examples of persons with various risk factors, their relative degrees of risk for developing cancer, and what they should do to modify those risks and thereby reduce their chance of developing cancer (and/or cardiovascular disease). After each risk factor the score is indicated in parentheses.

Consider the following. A 56-year-old (C) New Jersey (B) housewife (0) is 5 feet 5 inches tall, weighs 160 pounds (B), eats red meat daily, eats several eggs per week, drinks milk daily, consumes very little fiber-containing foods, and does not eat a balanced diet (A). She also smokes two packs of cigarettes a day, which she has done for over fifteen years (A). She drinks socially (0), has never had cancer (0), but her mother had breast cancer (B). She started having sexual intercourse at age 20 (0), first got pregnant at age 24 (0), has a history of fibrocystic breast disease (C), never had any radiation (0), and is relatively easygoing (0).

Her total score is 2 A's, 3 B's, and 2 C's. She is in the high-risk group. What can she do to modify her risk factors? She directly controls the most serious ones. I would advise her to terminate cigarette smoking abruptly and completely. Then I would suggest that she permanently modify her diet in order to reduce two other serious risk factors: her high-animal-fat, high-cholesterol, low-fiber diet, and her overweight problem. This would serve also to counter any weight gain that may occur when she stops smoking. She has no control over her age, the state in which she has lived, or her history of fibrocystic breast disease; but these are minor risk factors. By modifying the risk factors that she directly controls, over the course of time she will lessen her overall risk category and reduce her risk of developing cancer or cardiovascular disease.

The second example is a 24-year-old sexually active male homosexual who has many male partners and uses a drug called amyl nitrite (C). He smoked two packs of cigarettes a day for eleven years but quit one year ago (A). Up until a few months ago, he ate red meat daily, ate cheese daily, ate very few fiber-containing foods, and took no vitamins (A). His weight is normal (0), and he has never had cancer (0) nor have any of his family members (0). Until he was 21 years old he lived in Alaska (0), but he has since lived in New York City.

His total score is 2 A's, zero B's, and 1 C. He is in the high-risk group, but by continuing not to smoke and by modifying his diet he can dramatically lessen his overall risk.

Next is a 27-year-old woman who smoked two packs of cigarettes a day until she quit eight years ago (B). She eats a well-balanced diet consisting of red meat five times a week, low-fat dairy products, average intake of fiber (B), and she is 20 pounds overweight (C). As a lifelong resident of Vermont (C), she has been working in the furniture industry for the past seven years (B). She is taking birth control pills (B) and has been doing so for the past ten years. She is fair-skinned, sunburns easily, and enjoys sunbathing and using a suntanning booth year-round (B).

On the surface of things it looks as though her overall risk is not so bad, but when you examine the whole picture, you find she is in the moderate-risk category. Her total score is no A's, 5 B's, and 2 C's. However, she is on the right track. She should do the following to modify her risk factors and thereby reduce her overall risk: continue not to smoke, lose 20 pounds, modify her nutritional status, seek another means of birth control, use sun screens to sunbathe, and avoid suntanning boothes.

The last example is a 50-year-old (0) male chemist (B) who is 25 pounds overweight (B) and a meat-and-potatoes man all the way (A). He has smoked two packs of cigarettes a day for the past thirty years (A), drinks 4 ounces of whiskey every day (A), has lived in Illinois most of his life (B), and is easily angered (C). His father died of lung cancer (B).

You know that he is in the high-risk category: 3 A's, 4 B's, and 1 C. As you can see, he does have risk factors that he can directly control. He should do the following: stop smoking, drastically modify his diet and lose weight, consume alcohol in moderation, and learn how to relax. All these modifications will greatly reduce his overall risk.

You can now understand that with continued risk factor modification, your risk for developing cancer and heart disease will be greatly reduced. Modify those risk factors that you directly control. Remember, you must strive to achieve and maintain good health. Good health is no accident.

16

Diet Plan to Modify Risks

I WILL outline several easy-to-follow diets for weight reduction. Remember, it is not enough just to adhere to a good diet; you must also initiate some form of exercise, because you must use up more calories than you consume in order to lose weight. You must burn off 3500 calories to lose one pound. This means that if you are consuming 1000 calories per day and you burn off 1500 calories per day, you lose a total of 500 calories a day, and therefore it will take seven days to lose one pound. (See Table I in Chapter 8 for the effectiveness of different forms of exercise.) I recommend that initially you lose two to four pounds per week to get down to your ideal weight. Once you attain your weight goal you must modify your eating habits and life-style *permanently.* By adhering to the overall plan outlined in Chapter 15—eating a low-cholesterol, very low-fat, high-fiber diet, exercising moderately, and following all the other points listed—you will find that you will keep extra weight off and at the same time substantially reduce all risks for cancer and cardiovascular disease.

The types of food you eat are important, but often it is the amount of food that will determine your ultimate weight. Table I lists the six major food groups—milk, vegetable, fruit, meat and fish, bread, and fat—and Group 7 is miscellaneous. Starchy vegetables are listed in the bread group because, per

Table I

GROUP 1. MILK GROUP

Food	Serving	Cholesterol (mg)†	Calories	Fiber (gm)††
Cheeses:				
*American	1 oz	25	105	0
Cottage, 1% fat	½ cup	15	100	0
*Cheddar	1 oz	28	115	0
Monterey	1 oz	–	105	0
*Mozzarella	1 oz	30	80	0
Mozzarella, skim	1 oz	18	70	0
*Muenster	1 oz	25	105	0
Parmesan	1 oz	14	110	0
*Provolone	1 oz	28	100	0
Ricotta, skim	1 oz	14	171	0
*Swiss	1 oz	35	95	0
Cream:				
Light	1 tbs	10	32	0
*Half and half	1 tbs	6	20	0
*Heavy	1 tbs	20	53	0
*Ice cream, vanilla	½ cup	29	135	0
*Ice cream, chocolate	½ cup	30	140	0
Ice milk	½ cup	13	90	0
Milk, 2% fat	1 cup	22	120	0
Pudding: chocolate, vanilla, butterscotch, or banana made with 2% milk	½ cup	16	175	0
Sherbet	½ cup	–	135	0
Skim milk	1 cup	5	85	0
*Whole milk	1 cup	34	150	0
Yogurt, *whole milk,				
unflavored	1 cup	28	140	0
flavored	1 cup	24	250	0

Food	Serving	Cholesterol (mg)†	Calories	Fiber (gm)††
low-fat, unflavored	1 cup	17	125	0
flavored	1 cup	15	225	0

* These foods are to be avoided.

† Data for all food groups from Feeley, R. M., et al. 1972. Cholesterol content of food. *J. Am. Diet. Assoc.* 61:134.

†† Data for all food groups from McCance, R. A. and W. Widdowson. 1968. The composition of foods. London: Elsevier/North Holland Biomedical Press.

– Denotes no determined values.

GROUP 2. VEGETABLE GROUP

Food	Serving	Cholesterol (mg)	Calories	Fiber (gm)
Artichoke, cooked	1 bud	0	44	–
Asparagus	4 spears	0	10	.9
Asparagus, boiled, cut	½ cup	0	15	1.1
Avocado, fresh	½ whole	0	240	2.2
Bean sprouts	½ cup	0	5	1.6
Beets, boiled or sliced	½ cup	0	35	2.1
Broccoli, boiled & drained	½ cup	0	15	3.2
Brussels sprouts, boiled	½ cup	0	15	2.3
Cabbage, shredded, boiled	½ cup	0	10	2.0
Carrots, boiled, drained	½ cup	0	15	2.3
1 raw	7½"	0	20	2.3
Cauliflower, boiled, drained	½ cup	0	5	1.1
Celery, raw	1 stalk	0	5	.7
	½ cup	0	5	1.1
Coleslaw	½ cup	0	60	1.7
Cucumber, raw	6 slices	0	5	.1
1 small	6⅜"	0	5	.6
Dandelion green, cooked	½ cup	0	35	–
Eggplant, peeled and cooked	½ cup	0	15	2.5

Food	Serving	Cholesterol (mg)	Calories	Fiber (gm)
Green beans, boiled	½ cup	0	5	2.0
Green pepper	2 rings	0	5	0.2
1 medium	2¾″	0	15	0.8
Lettuce	⅙ head	0	10	1.4
	6 leaves	0	5	0.7
Mushrooms, raw	½ cup	0	5	0.9
Okra	½ cup	0	15	2.6
Onions, raw sliced	½ cup	0	15	0.7
boiled	½ cup	0	15	1.4
green	2 medium	0	10	0.9
Peas, boiled and drained	½ cup	0	40	4.2
Pickle, dill	3¾″ × 1¼″	0	5	1.1
Pumpkin	½ cup	0	40	0.5
Radishes	10 medium	0	10	0.5
Sauerkraut, solid and liquid	½ cup	0	20	3.3
Spinach, boiled and drained	½ cup	0	25	5.7
Tomato, raw	2½″	0	20	2.0
juice	½ cup	0	25	0
sauce	½ cup	0	115	2.6
Turnips, boiled and mashed	½ cup	0	15	3.2
Watercress, cut	½ cup	0	5	0.6
Zucchini	½ cup	0	15	–

GROUP 3. FRUIT GROUP

Food	Serving	Cholesterol (mg)	Calories	Fiber (gm)
Apple, with peel	2½″	0	50	2.1
Apple juice	⅓ cup	0	40	0
Applesauce, unsweetened	½ cup	0	40	2.6
Apricots	2	0	20	1.6

Food	Serving	Cholesterol (mg)	Calories	Fiber (gm)
Banana	½ small	0	40	1.6
Blackberries	½ cup	0	42	7.3
Blueberries	½ cup	0	45	–
Cantaloupe	¼	0	40	1.6
Cherries, sweet	10	0	30	1.2
Cranberries	½ cup	0	22	4.2
Dates, dried	2	0	18	0.8
Fig	1 medium	0	40	2.4
Fruit salad with syrup	¼ cup	0	60	1.4
Grapefruit, fresh	½ whole	0	20	0.6
canned, syrup packed	¼ cup	0	35	0.25
Grapefruit juice, sweet	⅓ cup	0	35	0.0
Grapes, seedless	12	0	20	0.3
Honeydew melon	$\frac{1}{10}$ melon	0	30	1.3
Lemon, fresh	1 slice	0	0	0.5
Lemon juice	1 tbs	0	5	0
Lemonade, frozen	¼ cup	0	30	0
Lychees	5	0	50	0.3
Mango	½	0	60	1.5
Nectarine	2½″	0	70	3.0
Olives	10	–	50	2.1
Orange	2½″	0	40	2.4
Orange juice	½ cup	0	55	0
Oranges, mandarin	½ cup	0	55	0.3
Papaya	½ of 3½″	0	60	–
Peach, fresh	2½″	0	35	1.4
canned, light syrup	¼ cup	0	35	0.6
Pear, fresh	2½″	0	45	2.6
Pineapple, fresh	½ cup	0	35	0.9
*canned, heavy syrup	¼ cup	0	50	0.6
juice, unsweetened	¼ cup	0	35	0
Plums, fresh	1″	0	10	0.4
Prunes, uncooked	2	0	20	2.0
stewed without sugar	½ cup	0	80	7.8
Raisins	2 tbs	0	45	1.2

Food	Serving	Cholesterol (mg)	Calories	Fiber (gm)
Raspberries	½ cup	0	15	4.6
Rhubarb, stewed with sugar	½ cup	0	55	2.8
Strawberries	½ cup	0	20	1.7
Tangerine	2½″	0	30	1.6
Watermelon	1 cup	0	40	–

GROUP 4. MEAT AND FISH GROUP

Food	Serving	Cholesterol (mg)	Calories	Fiber (gm)
Beef:				
Broth	1 cube	0	6	0
*Hamburger	3 oz	77	245	0
Pot pie, commercial	2 oz	9	109	0
*Rib roast	1 oz	26	69	0
Roast	1 oz	26	58	0
Flank steak, lean	1 oz	28	58	0
Vegetable stew, canned	1 cup	36	194	0
*Brains, raw	½ cup	2000	110	0
*Chicken, dark with skin	3 oz	82	150	0
*Chicken, white with skin	3 oz	69	140	0
Chicken pot pie, commercial	2 oz	8	125	0
Chicken, roasted, no skin:				
1 drumstick	1.3 oz	39	70	0
½ thigh	1 oz	24	48	0
¼ breast	1 oz	24	45	0
Chicken salad	⅓ cup	50	260	0.3
Egg:				
*Whole	1 large	252	82	0
White	1 large	0	17	0
*Yolk	1 large	252	72	0

Food	Serving	Cholesterol (mg)	Calories	Fiber (gm)
Fish:				
*Caviar, sturgeon	1 tbs	48	113	0
Clams	1 oz	14	21	0
Cod	1 oz	16	36	0
Crabs, steamed	2 oz	25	52	0
Flounder	1 oz	17	40	0
Haddock	1 oz	20	50	0
Halibut	1 oz	20	40	0
Herring	1 oz	30	75	0
Lobster, fresh	2 oz	31	54	0
Oysters, raw	1 oz	15	20	0
Salmon, broiled	2 oz	40	105	0
*Sardines, drained	1 oz	43	102	0
Scallops	1 oz	15	32	0
Shrimp, raw	1 oz	50	37	0
Trout	1 oz	20	40	0
*Tuna, in oil	2 oz	40	112	0
Tuna, in water	2 oz	32	70	0
Tuna salad	1 oz	18	70	0.5
Fish cakes	1 oz	–	55	0
Fish sticks, breaded	1 oz	–	70	0
*Hot dog	2 oz (1)	34	175	0
*Ham, boiled	3 oz	75	200	0
*Kidneys	8 oz	1125	90	0
$\frac{1}{3}$ Lamb chop	1 oz	30	55	0
Lamb, roast	1 oz	30	60	0
*Liver, beef	3 oz	372	150	0
*Liver, calf	3 oz	372	165	0
Meat loaf, lean	1 oz	28	55	0
Pork:				
$\frac{1}{3}$ chop	1 oz	25	80	0
*Loin	3 oz	72	215	0
*Sausage	1 link	34	60	0
Turkey, roasted, no skin:				
Dark meat	1 oz	30	60	0
White meat	1 oz	22	50	0
Turkey pot pie, commercial	2 oz	10	80	0
Veal cutlet, lean	1 oz	28	62	0

GROUP 5. BREAD GROUP

Food	Serving	Cholesterol (mg)	Calories	Fiber (gm)
Breads:				
Cracked wheat	1 slice	0	55	2.1
English muffin	½	0	50	0.9
Pumpernickel	1 slice	0	55	1.2
Raisin	1 slice	0	65	0.4
Rye	1 slice	0	60	1.2
White	1 slice	0	65	0.8
Whole wheat	1 slice	0	50	2.1
Dinner roll	1	0	75	0.8
Hot dog roll	½	0	60	0.6
Hamburger roll	½	0	60	0.6
Pancake, mix/egg/milk	4″ diameter	54	60	0.5
Taco shell	1	0	45	0
Waffle, mix/egg/milk	4″ diameter	60	61	0.6
Cereals and Grains:				
All-Bran	⅓ cup	0	70	9.0
40% Bran Flakes	⅓ cup	0	90	4.0
Cornflakes	⅓ cup	0	92	4.0
Grape-Nuts	⅓ cup	0	63	2.3
Puffed wheat	⅓ cup	0	104	5.1
Rice Krispies	⅓ cup	0	124	1.2
Shredded wheat	⅓ cup	0	108	4.1
Special K	⅓ cup	0	122	1.8
Sugar Puffs	⅓ cup	0	116	2.1
Corn flour	3½ oz	58	354	–
*Flour, white	3½ oz	–	337	3.0
Pasta:				
Noodles	3½ oz	101	100	–
Macaroni with cheese	3½ oz	21	370	–
Spaghetti with meat-balls/tomato sauce	3½ oz	75	378	–
Rice	3½ oz	2	361	2.4

Food	Serving	Cholesterol (mg)	Calories	Fiber (gm)
*Cakes:				
Angel food	$\frac{1}{12}$ 10″	0	120	0.1
Chocolate,				
chocolate frosting	$\frac{1}{16}$ 9″			
homemade		32	288	2.4
Box mix		33	294	2.4
Coffee cake	3″ x 2″ x 1$\frac{1}{2}$″	–	230	0.7
Cupcake, frosted	2$\frac{1}{2}$″	24	130	0.9
Fruitcake	2″ x 2″ x $\frac{1}{2}$″	7	115	3.4
Gingerbread	$\frac{1}{9}$ 8″	trace	373	1.3
Sponge cake	$\frac{1}{12}$ 12″	162	120	1.0
*Cookies:				
Brownies with nuts	1$\frac{3}{4}$″	17	128	–
Ladyfinger	4	157	170	0
*Pies				
Crackers:				
Rye wafers	3 3$\frac{1}{2}$″	0	65	2.3
Saltines	4	0	50	0
Vanilla wafers	4	0	75	0
Starchy vegetables:				
Baked beans	$\frac{1}{2}$ cup	–	95	11.0
Chili	$\frac{1}{2}$ cup	–	175	8.6
Corn: solid	$\frac{1}{3}$ cup	–	40	3.1
on the cob	1 ear	–	155	5.9
popped	1 cup	–	40	0.4
Potato: baked, with skin	2$\frac{1}{2}$″	–	130	3.0
boiled, peeled	2$\frac{1}{2}$″	–	105	2.7
mashed with milk	$\frac{1}{2}$ cup	–	125	0.9
sweet	5″ x 2 ″	–	130	3.5
Soups:				
Lentil, homemade	1 cup	–	240	5.5
Minestrone	1 cup	–	55	1.2

GROUP 6. FAT GROUP

Food	Serving	Cholesterol (mg)	Calories	Fiber (gm)
*Bacon, cooked and drained	1 strip	40	47	0
*Butter	1 pat (1 tsp)	35	35	0
Cheese sauce	¼ cup	14	130	0
Cooking or salad oil	1 tbs	–	120	0
Cream cheese	1 tbs	16	50	0
Dressings:				
French, low calorie	1 tbs	7	15	0
*French, regular	1 tbs	10	65	0
Italian, low calorie	1 tbs	6	10	0
*Italian, regular	1 tbs	9	85	0
*Margarine, animal/vegetable	1 pat (1 tsp)	35	102	0
Margarine, all-vegetable	1 pat (1 tsp)	0	35	0
Mayonnaise, low-calorie	1 tbs	5	47	0
Peanut butter, smooth	2 tbs	–	200	2.4
Peanuts, roasted and salted	¼ cup	–	205	2.9
Peanuts, Spanish	20	–	160	0.7
Sour cream	1 tbs	8	25	0
Tartar sauce, low-calorie	1 tbs	6	30	0
*Tartar sauce, regular	1 tbs	7	75	0
Walnuts: chopped	¼ cup	–	160	1.6
halves	¼ cup	–	130	1.3
White sauce	¼ cup	9	100	0

GROUP 7. MISCELLANEOUS

Food	Serving	Cholesterol (mg)	Calories	Fiber (gm)
Beverages:				
Alcoholic				
Beer, regular	12 oz	0	151	–
light	12 oz	0	96	–
Gin, rum, whiskey	$1\frac{1}{2}$ ounces			
80 proof		0	97	–
100 proof		0	124	–
Wines: dessert	4 oz	0	164	–
table	4 oz	0	100	–
Other beverages:				
Club soda	12 oz	0	0	0
Cola	12 oz	0	144	0
Cream soda	12 oz	0	160	0
Ginger ale	12 oz	0	113	0
Coffee	1 cup	0	2	0
Tea	1 cup	0	0	0
Gelatin	$\frac{1}{2}$ cup	–	70	0
*Honey	2 tbs	0	90	0
*Jelly	1 tsp	–	20	0
Ketchup	1 tbs	0	15	0
*Maple syrup	1 tbs	0	50	0
Mustard	1 tsp	–	5	0
*Sugar	1 tsp	0	15	0
Vinegar	1 tbs	0	0	0

serving, they contain the same amount of carbohydrate and protein as one slice of bread. In each group various foods are listed with their cholesterol content, calories, and fiber content, if known. In the recommended diets you will be able to "trade," or exchange, one food item for another in the same group; they are listed in portions that are approximately equivalent in calories and nutritional content. This trading will reduce the tediousness and take the chore out of dieting.

The foods of each group make a specific nutritional contribution. No one group can supply all the nutrients required for a well-balanced diet. However, the foods marked with an asterisk (*) are to be avoided because they have: (1) too high a total fat content (cholesterol is one component of the total fat content), or (2) too much concentrated sugar and may be too high in calories to be safe in your diet.

The grid below is an example of the way the diets are structured. This one is for dinner only. The numbers inside the grid represent the number of portions of a food in a particular group. One portion is the exact quantity listed under "Serving" in Table I. In the milk group (Group 1), you are allowed to take one half of the portion listed in Table I for skim milk, which turns out to be ½ cup. Next, you are allowed one portion of any food in the vegetable group (Group 2). Referring to Table I, this means that you could have 4 spears of asparagus, or ½ cup of bean sprouts, or ½ cup of green beans, and so on. Moving on, you are allowed one of any food in the fruit group (Group 3), again exactly as listed in the table. You can choose a small apple, half of a banana, half a grapefruit, ½ cup of fresh pineapple, ½ cup of raspberries, and so on. Next, you may eat three portions of any food listed in the meat group. That means you can have a chicken thigh and leg without skin, or 3 ounces of cod, or one whole pork chop, and so on. Nothing is listed in the bread or fat groups, so you cannot have any of these foods for this hypothetical dinner.

	Milk Group 1	Vegetable Group 2	Fruit Group 3	Meat Group 4	Bread Group 5	Fat Group 6
Breakfast						
Lunch						
Dinner	½ skim	1	1	3	—	—

In the box below, the approximate number of grams of protein, fat, and carbohydrate are given for one portion, or "trade," in the six major food groups. The total energy in calories for each portion is also shown. These values for calories are obtained by multiplying 4 times the number of grams of protein (1 gram of protein = 4 kcal), 9 times the number of grams of fat (1 gram of fat = 9 kcal), and 4 times the number of grams of carbohydrate (1 gram of carbohydrate = 4 kcal), and then adding up these answers for the total amount of calories for one portion. You can now see why you can lose much more weight and maintain that loss if you decrease the amount of fat in your diet, because there are over twice as many calories in 1 gram of fat as there are in either 1 gram of protein or 1 gram of carbohydrate.

While dieting to lose weight you should always:

1. Take a multiple vitamin/mineral complex daily.
2. Eat foods that are high in potassium, which include apricots, bananas, berries, grapefruit, grapefruit juice, mangoes, cantaloupes, honeydews, nectarines, oranges, orange juice, and peaches.
3. Remember, the more vegetables you eat the more gas you will have, because of the intestinal bacteria's action on the complex carbohydrates in vegetables. Don't despair, your

	Milk Group 1 portion	**Vegetable Group 1 portion**	**Fruit Group 1 portion**	**Meat Group 1 portion**	**Bread Group 1 portion**	**Fat Group 1 portion**
Protein	8 gr	2 gr	0	7 gr	2 gr	0
Fat	10 gr	0	0	5 gr	0	5 gr
Carbohydrate	12 gr	7 gr	10 gr	0	15 gr	0
Calories	170	36	40	73	68	45

system will adjust. The following *raw* vegetables may be used as desired: carrots, celery, chicory, Chinese cabbage, cucumbers, endive, escarole, lettuce, parsley, radishes, scallions, and watercress.

4. Look at the fiber content of the foods listed in Table I and try to choose a daily combination that will give you 12 to 15 grams of fiber. Choose cereals and breads with high fiber content. You can increase the fiber value of your breakfast by adding fruit to the cereal.

5. Drink as much water, bouillon without fat, and salt-free club soda as you desire. Consume tea and coffee in moderation—they do not have any calories, however.

6. Use freely the following seasonings: paprika, garlic, parsley, nutmeg, lemon, mustard, vinegar, mint, cinnamon, and lime. Use salt only while actually cooking. Do not use table salt.

Diets #1 and #2 contain approximately 1000 calories. You can see that the first diet has five meat trades and the second has four, but with an increase in vegetables and fruits. Either can be used, depending upon your taste for meat or vegetables. It also doesn't matter *when* you take the 5 meat trades in the first diet. For example, you may want one egg in the morn-

DIET # 1: 997.5 CALORIES PER DAY

	Milk Group 1	Vegetable Group 2	Fruit Group 3	Meat Group 4	Bread Group 5	Fat Group 6
Breakfast	1 skim		1		1	$\frac{1}{2}$
Lunch		2	2	2	1	
Dinner		2	1	3		

Protein: 55 grams per day
Fat: 37.5 grams per day
Carbohydrate: 110 grams per day

DIET # 2: 1000.5 CALORIES PER DAY

	Milk Group 1	Vegetable Group 2	Fruit Group 3	Meat Group 4	Bread Group 5	Fat Group 6
Breakfast	1 skim		1		1	½
Lunch		2	2	2	1	
Dinner		3	2	2		

Protein: 50 grams per day
Fat: 32.5 grams per day
Carbohydrate: 127 grams per day

ing, which then would leave 4 meat trades for the rest of the day. The same interchanging can be applied within any of the food groups of each diet; the breakfast/lunch/dinner designations aren't rigid.

Don't forget, these diets are designed only for weight loss, not maintenance. Once your weight goal is attained, you will have to increase the protein content somewhat in your daily diet. If you stick to these 1000-calorie-per-day diets *and* exercise you will lose a great deal of weight.

Diets #3 and #4 provide an additional 200 calories per day.

DIET # 3: 1218.5 CALORIES PER DAY

	Milk Group 1	Vegetable Group 2	Fruit Group 3	Meat Group 4	Bread Group 5	Fat Group 6
Breakfast	1 skim		1		1	½
Lunch		2	2	2	2	
Dinner		3	1	3	1	
Snack			1			

Protein: 61 grams per day
Fat: 37.5 grams per day
Carbohydrate: 157 grams per day

DIET # 4: 1255.5 CALORIES PER DAY

	Milk Group 1	Vegetable Group 2	Fruit Group 3	Meat Group 4	Bread Group 5	Fat Group 6
Breakfast	1 skim		1		1	$\frac{1}{2}$
Lunch		2	1	3	1	
Dinner		3	1	3	1	
Snack	$\frac{1}{2}$		1			

Protein: 70 grams per day
Fat: 47.5 grams per day
Carbohydrate: 138 grams per day

References

1. THE SCOPE OF CANCER

1. Bertino, J. R. 1977. Principles of neoplasia. *In:* Harrison's principles of internal medicine. Thorn, G. W., R. D. Adams, E. Braunwald, et al., eds. 8th ed. New York: McGraw-Hill.

2. Silverberg, E. 1983. Cancer statistics, 1983. *Ca-A Cancer J. for Clinicians* 33(1):9.

3. Rubin, P. 1978. Statement of the clinical oncological problem. *In:* Clinical oncology. Rubin, P., and R. F. Bakemeier, eds. 5th ed. New York: American Cancer Society, Inc.

4. Silverberg. Cancer statistics.

5. U.S. National Center for Health Statistics and the U.S. Bureau of the Census. 1980.

6. Atlas of Cancer Mortality in the Peoples' Republic of China. China Map Press. 1982. Edited by the Editorial Committee for the Atlas.

2. RISK FACTORS

1. The National Academy of Sciences. 1982. Nutrition, diet, and cancer.

2. Wynder, E. L., and G. B. Gori. 1977. Contribution of the environment to cancer incidence: an epidemiologic exercise. *J. Natl. Cancer Inst.* 58:825.

3. Workshop on Fat and Cancer. September 1981. Supplement to *Cancer Res.* 41(9):3677.

4. Mulvihill, J. J. 1977. Genetic repertory of human neoplasia. *In:* Genetics of human cancer. Mulvihill, J. J., R. W. Miller, and J. F. Fraumeni, eds. New York: Raven Press, 137.

5. Armstrong, B., and R. Doll. 1975. Environmental factors and cancer incidence and mortality in different countries, with special reference to dietary practices. *Intl. J. Cancer* 15:617.

6. Bjarnason, O., N. Day, G. Snaedal, and H. Tilinuis. 1974. The effect

of year of birth on the breast cancer age incidence curve in Iceland. *Intl. J. Cancer* 13:689.

7. Miller, A. B. 1980. Nutrition and cancer. *Prev. Med.* 9:189.

8. Eskin, B. A. 1978. Iodine and mammary cancer. *In:* Inorganic and Nutritional Aspects of Cancer. G. H. Schrauzer, ed. New York: Plenum Press, 293–304.

9. Upton, A. C. 1980. Future directions in cancer prevention. *Prev. Med.* 9:309.

10. Alpert, M. E., M. S. R. Hutt, G. N. Wogan, et al. 1971. Association between aflatoxin content of food and hepatoma frequency in Uganda. *Cancer* 28:253.

11. Shank, R. C., G. N. Wogan, J. B. Gibson, et al. 1972. Dietary aflatoxins and human liver cancer. II. Aflatoxins in market foods and foodstuffs of Thailand and Hong Kong. *Food Cosmet. Toxicol.* 10:61.

12. MacMahon, B., S. Yen, D. Trichopoulos, et al. 1981. Coffee and cancer of the pancreas. *New Eng. J. Med.* 304:630.

13. Feinstein, A. R., R. I. Horwitz, W. O. Spitzer, and R. N. Battista. 1981. Coffee and pancreatic cancer. *JAMA* 246:957.

14. Goldstein, H. R. 1982. No association found between coffee and cancer of the pancreas. *N. Eng. J. Med.* 306:997.

15. Tomatis, L., C. Agthe, H. Bartsch, et al. 1978. Evaluation of the carcinogenicity of chemicals: A review of the monograph program of the International Agency for Research on Cancer. *Cancer Res.* 38:877.

16. Wattenberg, L. W. 1978. Inhibitors of chemical carcinogenesis. *Adv. Cancer Res.* 26:197.

17. International Agency for Research on Cancer. 1980. Annual Report. World Health Organization. Lyon, France.

18. Fox, A. J., E. Lynge, and H. Malker. 1982. Lung cancer in butchers. *Lancet* i:156.

19. Johnson, E. S., and H. R. Fischman. 1982. Cancer mortality among butchers and slaughterhouse workers. *Lancet* i:913.

20. Miller, D. G. 1980. On the nature of susceptibility to cancer. *Cancer* 46:1307.

21. Walford, R. L. 1969. The immunological theory of aging. Munksgaard, Copenhagen.

22. Kahn, H. A. 1966. The Dorn study of smoking and mortality among U.S. veterans: Report on eight and one-half years of observation. *In:* Epidemiological study of cancer and other chronic diseases. Natl. Cancer Inst. Mono. 19. Washington, D.C. U.S. Government Printing Office. 1.

23. Ibid.

24. Benditt, E. P., and J. M. Benditt. 1973. Evidence for a monoclonal origin of human atherosclerotic plaques. *Proc. Natl. Acad. Sci. USA.* 70:1753.

25. Shu, H. P., and A. V. Nichols. 1979. Benzo(a)pyrene uptake by human plasma lipoproteins *in vitro. Cancer Res.* 39:1224.

26. Pero, R. W., C. Bryngelsson, F. Mitelman, et al. 1976. High blood pressure related to carcinogen induced unscheduled DNA synthesis, DNA carcinogen binding, and chromosomal aberrations in human lymphocytes. *Proc. Natl. Acad. Sci. USA.* 73:2496.

27. de Waard, F., E. A. Banders-van Halewijn, and J. Huizinga. 1964. The bimodal age distribution of patients with mammary cancer. *Cancer* 17:141.

28. Dyer, A. R., J. Stamler, A. M. Berkson, et al. 1975. High blood pressure: A risk factor for cancer mortality. *Lancet* 1:1051.

29. Paffenbarger, R. S., E. Fasal, M. E. Simmons, et al. 1977. Cancer risk as related to use of oral contraceptives during fertile years. *Cancer Res.* 39:1887.

30. Pike, M. C., H. A. Edmondson, B. Benton, et al. 1977. *In:* Origins of human cancer. Book A. Incidence of cancer in humans. Cold Spring Harbor Lab., 423–27.

31. Wobbes, T., H. S. Koops, and J. Oldhoff. 1980. The relation between testicular tumors, undescended testes, and inguinal hernias. *J. Surg. Onc.* 14:45.

32. Armstrong and Doll. Environmental factors.

33. Bjarnason, Day, et al. Effect of year of birth.

34. de Waard, F. 1975. Breast cancer incidence and nutritional status with particular reference to body weight and height. *Cancer Res.* 35:3351.

35. Gray, G. E., M. C. Pike, and B. E. Henderson. 1979. Breast cancer incidence and mortality rates in different countries in relation to known risk factors and dietary practices. *Br. J. Cancer* 39:1.

36. Miller, A. B. 1978. An overview of hormone-associated cancers. *Cancer Res.* 38:3985.

37. Monson, R. R., S. Yen, and B. MacMahon. 1976. Chronic mastitis and carcinoma of the breast. *Lancet* 2:224.

38. Leis, H. P., C. S. Kwon. 1979. Fibrocystic diseases of the breast. *J. Reprod. Med.* 22:291.

39. Narayana, A. S., et al. 1982. Carcinoma of the penis. *Cancer* 49:2185.

40. Hymes, K. B., et al. 1981. Kaposi's sarcoma in homosexual men—a report of eight cases. *Lancet* 19:598.

41. Thomsen, H. K., et al. 1981. Kaposi's sarcoma among homosexual men in Europe. *Lancet* 21:688.

42. Goedert, J. J., et al. 1982. Amyl nitrite may alter T lymphocytes in homosexual men. *Lancet* 20:412.

43. Gottleib, M. S., et al. 1981. *Pneumocystis carinii* pneumonia and mucosal candidiasis in previously healthy homosexual men. *N. Eng. J. Med.* 305:1425.

44. Siegal, F. P., et al. 1981. Severe acquired immunodeficiency in male homosexuals, manifested by chronic perianal ulcerative herpes simplex lesions. *N. Eng. J. Med.* 305:1439.

45. Goedert et al. Amyl nitrite.

46. Wallace, J. I., et al. 1982. T cell ratios in homosexuals. *Lancet* 17:908.

47. Daling, J. R., et al. 1982. Correlates of homosexual behavior and the incidence of anal cancer. *JAMA* 247:1988.

48. Pierce, R. C., and M. Katz. 1975. Dependency of polynuclear aromatic hydrocarbons on size distribution of atmospheric aerosols. *Environ. Sci. Technol.* 9:347.

49. U.S. Environmental Protection Agency. 1975a. Preliminary assessment of suspected carcinogens in drinking water. Report to Congress. Environmental Protection Agency, Washington, D.C.

50. Harris, R. H., T. Page, and N. A. Reiches. 1977b. Carcinogenic hazards of organic chemicals in drinking water. *In:* Hiatt, H. H., et al., eds. Book A. Incidence of cancer in humans. Cold Spring Harbor Lab.

3. THE BACKBONE OF NUTRITION

1. Brock, J. F., and M. Autret. 1952. Kwashiorkor in Africa. WHO Monograph Series. No. 8. Geneva: WHO.

2. Consalazio, C. F., H. L. Johnson, R. A. Nelson, J. G. Dramise, and J. H. Shala. 1975. Protein metabolism during intensive physical training in the young adult. *Am. J. Clin. Nutr.* 28:29.

3. Harrison, F. C., and A. D. King-Roach. 1976. Cell size and glucose oxidation rate in adipose tissue from non-diabetic and diabetic obese human subjects. *Clin. Sci. Mol. Med.* 50:171.

4. NUTRITION, IMMUNITY, AND CANCER

1. Cannon, P. R. 1942. Antibodies and protein reserves. *J. Immunol.* 44:107.

2. Rous, P. 1914. The influence of diet on transplanted and spontaneous mouse tumors. *J. Exp. Med.* 20:433.

3. Tannenbaum, A. 1940. The initiation and growth of tumors. Introduction I. Effects of underfeeding. *Am. J. Cancer* 38:335.

4. Simone, C. B., and P. A. Henkart. 1980. Permeability changes induced in erythrocyte ghost targets by antibody-dependent cytotoxic effector cells: Evidence for membrane pores. *J. Immunol.* 124:954.

5. Burnet, F. M. 1970. Immunological surveillance. Oxford: Pergamon Press.

6. Kersey, J. H., G. D. Spector, and R. A. Good. 1973. Primary immunodeficiency diseases and cancer: The immunodeficiency-cancer registry. *Intl. J. Cancer* 12:333.

7. Spector, G. D., G. S. Perry III, R. A. Good, and J. H. Kersey. 1978. Immunodeficiency diseases and malignancy. *In:* The immunopathology of lymphoreticular neoplasms. Twomey, J. J., and R. A. Good, eds. New York: Plenum Publishing, 203.

8. Penn, I. 1970. *In:* Malignant tumors in organ transplant recipients. New York: Springer-Verlag.

9. Birkeland, S. A., E. Kemp, and M. Hauge. 1975. Renal transplantation and cancer. The Scandia transplant material. *Tissue Antigens* 6:28.

10. Aschekenasy, A. 1975. Dietary protein and amino acids in leucopoiesis. *World Rev. Nutri. Diet* 21:152.

11. Jose, D. G., and R. A. Good. 1971. Absence of enhancing antibody in cell-mediated immunity to tumor homografts in protein deficient rats. *Nature* 231:807.

12. Passwell, J. H., M. W. Steward, and J. F. Soothill. 1974. The effects of protein malnutrition on macrophage function and the amount and affinity of antibody response. *Clin. Exp. Immunol.* 17:491.

13. Van Oss, C. J. 1971. Influence of glucose levels on the *in vitro* phagocytosis of bacteria by human neutrophils. *Infect. Immunol.* 4:54.

14. Perille, P. E., J. P. Nolan, and S. C. Finch. 1972. Studies of the resistance to infection in diabetes mellitus: local exudative cellular response. *J. Lab. Clin. Med.* 59:1008.

15. Bagdade, J. D., R. K. Root, and R. J. Bulger. 1974. Impaired leukocyte function in patients with poorly controlled diabetes. *Diabetes* 23:9.

16. Stuart, A. E., and A. E. Davidson. 1976. Effect of simple lipids on antibody formation after ingestion of foreign red cells. *J. Pathol. Bacteriol.* 87:305.

17. Santiago-Delpin, E. A., and J. Szepsenwol. 1977. Prolonged survival of skin and tumor allografts in mice on high fat diets. *J. Natl. Cancer Inst.* 59:459.

18. DiLuzio, N. R., and W. R. Wooles. 1964. Depression of phagocytic activity and immune response by methyl palmitate. *Am. J. Physiol.* 206:939.

19. Clausen, J., and J. Moller. 1969. Allergic encephalomyelitis induced by brain antigen after deficiency in polyunsaturated fatty acids during myelination. *Int. Arch. Allergy Appl. Immunol.* 36:224.

20. Meade, C. J., and J. Mertin. 1976. The mechanism of immunoinhibition by arachidonic and linoleic acid. Effects on the lymphoid and RE systems. *Int. Arch. Allergy Appl. Immunol.* 51:2.

5. FREE RADICALS

1. Weves, R., D. Roos, R. S. Weening, et al. 1976. An EPR study of myeloperoxidase in human granulocytes. *Biochim. Biophys. Acta.* 421:328.

2. Tam, B. K., and P. B. McKay. 1970. Reduced triphosphopyridine nucleotide oxidase-catalysed alterations of membrane phospholipids, III. Transient formation of phospholipid peroxides. *J. Biol. Che.* 245:2295.

3. Reich, L., and S. S. Stivala. 1969. *In:* Autoxidation of hydrocarbons and polyoletins. New York: Dekker.

4. Lundberg, W. O. 1961. *In:* Autoxidation and antioxidants. Vol. I. New York: Wiley.

5. Pryor, W. A. 1971. Background radiation. *Chem. Eng. News.* 49:34.

6. Wills, E. D. 1970. *Int. J. Rad. Res.* 17:229.

7. Norins, A. L. 1962. Free radical formation in skin following exposure to ultraviolet light. *J. Invest. Dermatol.* 39:445.

8. Urbach, F., J. H. Epstein, and P. D. Forbes. 1974. *In:* Sunlight and man. Pathak, M. A., et al., eds. Tokyo: Univ. Tokyo Press, 259.

9. Zelac, R. E., H. L. Cromroy, W. E. Bloch, et al. 1971. Inhaled ozone as a mutagen. I. Chromosome aberration induced in Chinese hamster lymphocytes. *Environ. Res.* 4:262.

10. Pryor, W. A. 1973. Free radical reactions and their importance in biochemical systems. *Fed. Proc., Fed. Amer. Soc. Exp. Biol.* 32:1862.

11. Slater, T. F. 1972. *In:* Free radical mechanism in tissue injury. London. Pion, Ltd.

12. Recknagel, R. O. 1967. Carbon tetrachloride hepatoxicity. *Pharmacol. Rev.* 19:145.

13. Fridovich, I. 1975. Superoxide dismutases. *Ann. Rev. Biochem.* 44:147.

14. Ogura, Y. 1955. Catalase activity at high concentrations of hydrogen peroxide. *Arch. Biophys.* 57:228.

15. Christopherson, B. O. 1969. Reduction of linoleic acid hydroperoxide by a glutathione peroxidase. *Biochem. Biophys. Acta.* 176:463.

16. Wattenberg, W. L., W. O. Loub, L. K. Lam, and J. L. Speier. 1976. Dietary constituents altering the response to chemical carcinogens. *Fed. Proc.* 35:1327.

6. VITAMINS AND MINERALS

1. Leevy, C. M., L. Cardi, O. Frank, et al. 1965. Incidence and significance of hypovitaminemia in a randomly selected municipal hospital population. *Am. J. Clin. Nutr.* 17:259.

1a. Peto, R., R. Doll, J. D. Buckley, and M. B. Sporn. 1981. Can dietary beta-carotene materially reduce human cancer rates? *Nature* 290:201.

1b. World Health Organization. 1974. Technical Report. Ser. No. 557.

2. Meltzer, M. S., and B. E. Cohen. 1974. Tumor regression by Mycobaterium-bovis (strain BCG) enhanced by vitamin A. *J. Natl. Cancer Inst.* 53:585.

3. Kurata, T., and M. Micksche. 1977. Immunoprophalaxis in Lewis lung tumor with vitamin A and BCG. *Sci.* 5:277.

4. Lotan, R. 1979. Different susceptibilities of human melanoma and breast carcinoma cell lines to retinoic acid-induced growth inhibition. *Cancer Res.* 39:1014.

5. Ibid.

6. Micksche, M., C. Cerni, O. Kokron, et al. 1977. Stimulation of immune response in lung cancer patients by vitamin A therapy. *Oncology* 34:234.

7. Mettlin, C., S. Graham, and M. Swanson. 1979. Vitamin A and lung cancer. *J. Nat. Cancer Inst.* 62:1435.

8. Krishnan, S., U. N. Bhuyan, et al. 1974. Effect of vitamin A and protein calories undernutrition on immune response. *Immunol.* 27:383.

9. Genta, V. M., D. G. Kaufmann, C. C. Harris, et al. 1974. Vitamin A deficiency enhances binding of benzo(a)pyrene to tracheal epithelial DNA. *Nature* 247:48.

10. Rosenberg, H., and A. N. Felzman. 1974. *In:* The book of vitamin therapy. New York: Berkley Publishing Corp.

11. Goodman, L. S., and A. Gilman, eds. 1977. *In:* A pharmacological basis of therapeutics. 5th ed. New York: Macmillan.

12. Rosenberg and Felzman. *In:* Book of vitamin therapy.

13. Jaffe, W. 1946. The influence of wheat germ on the production of tumors in rats by methylcholanthrene. *Exp. Med. Surg.* 4:278.

14. Haber, S. L., and R. W. Wissler. 1962. Effect of vitamin E on carcinogenicity of methylcholanthrene. *Proc. Soc. Exp. Biol. Med.* 111:774.

15. Harman, D. 1969. Dibenzanthracene induced cancer: Inhibition effect of dietary vitamin E. *Clin. Res.* 17:125.

16. Monson, R. R., S. Yen, and B. MacMahon. 1976. Chronic mastitis and carcinoma of the breast. *Lancet* 2:224.

17. Leis, H. P., and C. S. Kwon. 1979. Fibrocystic disease of the breast. *J. Reprod. Med.* 22:291.

18. London, R., D. Solomon, E. London, et al. 1978. Mammary dysplasia: Clinical response and urinary excretion of 11-desoxy 17 keto-steroids and pregnandiol following alpha-tocopherol therapy. *Breast, Diseases of the Breast* 4(2):19.

19. London, R., G. S. Sundaram, M. Schultz, et al. 1981. Alpha-tocopherol, mammary dysplasia and steroid hormones. *Cancer Res.* In press.

20. Guggenheim, K., and E. Buechler. 1946. Thiamine deficiency and susceptibility of rats and mice to infection with Salmonella typhimurium. *Proc. Soc. Exp. Biol. Med.* 61:413.

21. Morgan, A. F., M. Groody, and H. E. Axelrod. 1946. Pyridoxine deficiency in dogs as affected by level of dietary protein. *Am. J. Physiol.* 146:723.

22. Ibid.

23. Robson, L. C., and M. R. Schwarz. 1975. Vitamin B_6 deficiency and the lymphoid system. I. Effects on cellular immunity and *in vitro* incorporation of ^{3}H-uridine by small lymphocytes. *Cell. Immunol.* 16:145.

24. Kamm, J. J., T. Dashman, A. H. Conney, and J. J. Burns. 1973. Protective effects of ascorbic acid on hepatotoxicity caused by sodium nitrite plus aminopyrine. *Proc. Natl. Acad. Sci.* 70:743.

25. Weisburger, J. H. 1979. Mechanism of action of diet as a carcinogen. *Cancer* 43:1987.

26. Pipkin, G. E., R. Nishimura, L. Banowsky, and J. U. Schlegel. 1967. Stabilization of urinary 3 hydroxyanthranilic acid by oral administration of L-ascorbic acid. *Proc. Soc. Exp. Biol. Med.* 126:702.

27. Schlegel, J. U. 1975. Proposed uses of ascorbic acid in prevention of bladder carcinoma. *Ann. N.Y. Acad. Sci.* 258:423.

28. Gluttenplan, J. B. 1978. Mechanism of inhibition of ascorbate of microbial mutagenesis induced by N-nitroso compounds. *Cancer Res.* 38:2018.

29. Pauling, L. 1972. Preventive nutrition. *Medicine on the Midway* 27:15.

30. Cameron, E. 1966. *In:* Hyaluronidase and cancer. New York. Pergamon Press.

31. Herbert, V. D. 1977. *Contemp. Nutr.* 2(10).

32. Hoffer, A. 1971. Ascorbic acid and toxicity. *N. Eng. J. Med.* 285:635.

33. Klenner, F. R. 1971. Vitamin C and toxicity. *J. Appl. Nutr.* 23:61.

34. Schrauzer, G. N., and D. A. White. 1978. Selenium in human nutrition: Dietary intakes and effects of supplementation. *Bioinorganic Chem.* 8:303.

35. Schrauzer, G. N., D. A. White, and C. J. Sneider. 1977. Cancer mortality correlation studies. III. Statistical associations with dietary selenium intakes. *Bioinorganic Chem.* 7:23–34, 35–56.

36. Shamberger, R. J. 1966. Protection against cocarcinogenesis by antioxidants. *Experientia.* 22:116.

37. Shamberger, R. J., and C. Willis. 1971. Selenium distribution and human cancer mortality. *Clin. Lab. Sci.* 2:211.

38. Ibid.

39. Ip, C., D. K. Sinha. 1981. Enhancement of mammary tumorigenesis by dietary selenium deficiency in rats with a high polyunsaturated fat intake. *Cancer Res.* 41:31.

40. Medina, R., et al. 1981. Editorial. Selenium may act as cancer inhibitor. *JAMA* 246:1510.

41. Kurkela, P. 1977. The health of Finnish diet. 22nd Gen. Conf. Internat. Fed. of Agricultural Producers. Helsinki, Finland.

42. Chinese Academy of Medical Sciences. 1977. Keshan Disease Group. Beijing. Epidemiologic studies on the etiologic relationship of selenium and Keshan disease. *Chin. Med. J.* 92:477.

43. Schrauzer, White, and Sneider. Cancer mortality.

44. Young, V. R., and D. Richardson. 1979. Nutrients, vitamins, and minerals in cancer prevention. Facts and fallacies. *Cancer* 43:2125.

45. Sakurai, H. and K. Tsuchiya. 1975. A tentative recommendation for the maximum daily intake of selenium. *Environ. Physiol. Biochem.* 5:107.

46. Danbolt, N., and K. Closs. 1942. Akrodermatitis enteropathica. *Acta. Derm. Venereol.* 23:127.

47. Good, R. A., G. Fernandes, et al. 1979. Nutrition, immunity, and cancer—a review. *Clin. Bull.* 9:3–12, 63–75.

48. McMahon, L. J., D. W. Montgomery, A. Guschewsky, et al. 1976. *In vitro* effects of $ZnCl_2$ on spontaneous sheep red blood cells (E) rosette formation by lymphocytes from cancer patients and normal subjects. *Immunol. Commun.* 5:53.

49. Frost, P., J. C. Chen, I. Rabbini, et al. 1977. The effects of zinc deficiency on the immune response. *Proc. Clin. Biol. Res.* 14:143.

50. Lennard, E. S., A. B. Bjornson, et al. 1974. An immunologic and nutritional evaluation of burn neutrophil functions. *J. Surg. Res.* 16:286.

51. Basu, T. K. 1976. Significance of vitamins in cancer. *Oncology* 33:183.

52. Bertino, J. R. 1979. Nutrients, vitamins, and minerals as therapy. *Cancer* 43:2137.

7. FOOD ADDITIVES AND CONTAMINANTS

1. Resin, A., and H. Ungar. 1957. Malignant tumors in the eyelids and the auricular region of thiourea treated rats. *Cancer Res.* 17:302.

2. Nelson, A. A., and G. Woodard. 1953. Tumors of the urinary bladder, gall bladder, and liver in dogs fed o-aminoazotoluene or p dimethyl aminoazobenzene. *J. Nat. Cancer Inst.* 13:1497.

3. Witschi, H., D. Williamson, and S. Lock. 1977. Enhancement of urethan tumorigenesis in mouse lung by butylated hydroxytoluene. *J. Nat. Cancer Inst.* 58:301.

4. Wattenberg, L. W. 1978. Inhibition of chemical carcinogenesis. *J. Nat. Cancer Inst.* 60:11.

5. Munro, E. C., C. Moodie, D. Krewski, et al. 1975. A carcinogenicity study of commercial saccharin in the rat. *Toxicol. Appl. Pharmacol.* 32:513.

6. Kessler, I. 1976. Non-nutritive sweeteners and human bladder cancer: Preliminary findings. *J. Urol.* 115:143.

7. Shubik, P. 1979. Food additives (natural and synthetic). *Cancer* 43: 1982.

8. Sen, N. P. 1972. The evidence for the presence of dimethylnitrosamine in meat products. *Food Cosmet. Toxicol.* 10:219.

9. Newberne, P. M. 1979. Nitrite promotes lymphoma incidence in rats. *Science* 204:1079.

10. Shubik, P. 1980. Food additives, contaminants, and cancer. *Prev. Med.* 9:197.

11. Toth, B., and D. Nagel. 1978. Tumors induced in mice by N-methyl-N-formylhydrazine of the false moral *Gyromitra esculenta. J. Nat. Cancer Inst.* 60:201.

12. Lijinsky, W., and P. Shubik. 1964. Benzo(a)pyrene and other polynuclear hydrocarbons in charcoal broiled meats. *Science* 145:53.

13. Ibid.

8. OBESITY

1. Hannon, B. M., and T. G. Lohman. 1978. The energy cost of overweight in the United States. *Am. J. Public Health* 68:8.

2. McCay, C. M., M. F. Crowell, and L. A. Maynard. 1935. The effect of retarded growth upon the length of lifespan and upon the ultimate size. *J. Nutr.* 10:63.

3. Jose, D. G., and R. A. Good. 1973. Quantitative effects of nutritional protein and caloric deficiency upon the immune response to tumors in mice. *Cancer Res.* 33:807.

4. Jose, D. G., O. Stutman, and R. A. Good. 1973. Good, long term effects on immune function of early nutritional deprivation. *Nature* 241:57.

5. Tannenbaum, A. 1959. Nutrition and cancer. *In:* Physiopathy of cancer. Homberger, F., ed. 2nd ed. New York: Hoeber-Harper, 517–62.

6. Kraybill, H. F. 1963. Carcinogenesis associated with foods, food additives, food degradation products and related dietary factors. *Clin. Pharmacol. Ther.* 4:73.

7. Jose and Good. Quantitative effects.

8. Drori, D., and Y. Folman. 1976. Environmental effects on longevity in the male rat: exercise, mating, castration, and restricted feeding. *Exp. Gerontol.* 11:25.

9. Ross, M. H., and G. Bras. 1971. Lasting influence of early caloric restriction on prevalence of neoplasms in the rat. *J. Natl. Cancer Inst.* 47:1095.

10. National Dairy Council. 1975. Nutrition, diet, and cancer. *Dairy Council Digest* 46(5):25.

11. Gaskill, S. P., W. L. McGuire, et al. 1979. Breast cancer mortality and diet in the United States. *Cancer Res.* 39:3628.

12. Sylvester, P. W., et al. 1981. Relationship of hormones to inhibition of mammary tumor development by underfeeding during the "critical period" after carcinogen administration. *Cancer Res.* 41:1384.

13. Newberne, P. M., and G. Williams. 1979. Nutritional influences on the cause of infection. *In:* Resistance to infectious diseases. Dunlop, R. H., and H. W. Moon, eds. Saskatoon: Saskatoon Modern Press.

14. Leonard, P. J. and K. M. MacWilliam. 1964. Cortisol binding in the serum in kwashiorkor. *J. Endocrinol.* 29:273.

9. SMOKING

1. Public Health Service. 1979. Smoking and health, a report of the surgeon general. U.S. Dept. of HEW.

2. Shackney, S. E. 1982. Carcinogenesis and tumor cell biology. 1982 Surgeon General's Report.

3. Hirayama, T. 1979. Diet and cancer. *Nutrition and Cancer* 1(3):67.

4. Winn, D. M., W. J. Blot, et al. 1981. Snuff dipping and oral cancer among women in the southern United States. *New Eng. J. Med.* 304:745.

5. Pic, A. 1981. Heavy smoking and exercise can trigger MI. *Int. Med. News.* 14(9):3.

6. Hopkin, J. M., and H. J. Evans. 1980. Cigarette smoke induced DNA damage and lung cancer risks. *Nature* 283:388.

7. Evans, H. J., et al. 1981. Sperm abnormalities and cigarette smoking. *Lancet* (March):627.

8. Repace, J. L. 1981. The problems of passive smoking. *Bull. N.Y. Acad. Med.* 57(10):936.

9. Hirayama, T. 1981. Non-smoking wives of heavy smokers have a higher risk of lung cancer: a study from Japan. *Br. Med. J.* 282:163.

10. White, J. R., and H. F. Froeb. 1980. Small airways dysfunction in nonsmokers chronically exposed to tobacco smoke. *New Eng. J. Med.* 302:720.

10. ALCOHOL AND CAFFEINE

1. Shaw, S., and C. S. Lieber. 1977. Alcoholism. *In:* Nutritional support of medical practice. New York: Harper and Row, 202–21.

2. Rosenberg, L., D. Sloan, S. Shapiro, et al. 1982. Breast cancer and alcoholic consumption. *Lancet* 30:267.

3. Lundy, J., et al. 1975. The acute and chronic effects of alcohol on the human immune system. *Surg. Gyn. Obst.* 141:212.

4. Simon, D., S. Yen, and P. Cole. 1975. Coffee drinking and cancer of the lower urinary tract system. *J. Natl. Cancer Inst.* 54(3):587.

5. Mulvihill, J. 1973. Caffeine as teratogen and mutagen. *Teratology* 8:69.

6. Weinstein, D., I. Mauer, and H. Solomon. 1972. The effects of caffeine on chromosomes of human lymphocytes. *Mutat. Res.* 16:391.

7. Soyka, L. F. 1979. Effects of methylxanthines on the fetus. *Clinics in Perinatol.* 6(1):37.

8. Weathersbee, P. S., L. K. Olsen, and J. R. Lodge. 1977. Caffeine and pregnancy. *Postgrad. Med.* 62(3):64.

II. BREAST CANCER

1. National Cancer Institute. 1977. *In:* Cancer patient survival report. No. 5, 1976. DHEW Publication No. (NIH) 77–992. Bethesda, Md.: N.C.I.

2. Alcantara, E. N., and E. W. Speckman. 1976. Diet, nutrition, and cancer. *Am. J. Clin. Nutr.* 29:1035.

3. Carroll, K. K. 1975. Experimental evidence of dietary factors and hormone dependent cancers. *Cancer Res.* 35:3374.

4. Wynder, E. L. 1979. Dietary habits and cancer epidemiology. *Cancer* 43:1955.

5. Tannenbaum, A. 1942. The genesis and growth of tumors. III. Effects of a high fat diet. *Cancer Res.* 2:468.

6. Carroll, K. K., E. B. Gammel, and E. R. Plunkett. 1968. Dietary fat and mammary cancer. *Can. Med. Assoc. J.* 98:590.

7. Drasar, B. S., and D. Irving. 1973. Environmental factors and cancer of the colon and breast. *Br. J. Cancer* 27:167.

8. Hems, G. 1970. Epidemiologic characteristics of breast cancer in middle and late age. *Br. J. Cancer.* 24:226.

9. Phillips, R. L. 1975. Role of life-style and dietary habits in risk of cancer among Seventh-Day Adventists. *Cancer Res.* 35:3513.

10. Kent, S. 1979. Diet, hormones, and breast cancer. *Geriatrics* 34:83.

11. Haenzel, W., et al. 1973. Large bowel cancer in Hawaiian Japanese. *J. Natl. Cancer Inst.* 51:1765.

12. Gaskill, S. P., et al. 1979. Breast cancer mortality and diet in the United States. *Cancer Res.* 39:3628.

13. Reddy, B. S., A. Mastromarino, and E. Wynder. 1977. Diet and metabolism: large bowel cancer. *Cancer* 39:1815.

14. Reddy, B. S., and E. Wynder. 1977. Metabolic epidemiology of colon cancer. *Cancer* 39:2533.

15. Paptestas, A. E., et al. 1982. Fecal steroid metabolites and breast cancer risk. *Cancer* 49:1201.

16. Brammer, S. H. and R. L. DeFelice. 1980. Dietary advice in regard to risk for colon and breast cancer. *Prev. Med.* 9:544.

17. Chan, P. C., J. F. Head, L. A. Cohen, et al. 1977. Effect of high fat diet on serum prolactin levels and mammary cancer development in ovariectomized rats. *Proc. Am. Assoc. Cancer Res.* 18:189.

18. Brammer and DeFelice. Dietary advice.

19. Petrakis, N. L., L. D. Gruenke, and J. C. Craig. 1981. Cholesterol and cholesterol epoxide in nipple aspirate of human breast fluid. *Cancer Res.* 41:2563.

20. Wynder. Dietary habits.

21. Schwarz, B. E. 1981. Does estrogen cause adenocarcinoma of the endometrium? *Clin. Obst. Gyn.* 24:243.

22. Orentreich, N., and N. P. Durr. 1974. Mammogenesis in transsexuals. *J. Invest. Dermatol.* 63:142.

23. Symmers, W. S. 1968. Carcinoma of the breast in transsexuals. *Br. Med. J.* 1:83.

24. Treves, N., and A. Hollcb. 1955. Cancer of the male breast. *Cancer* 8:1239.

25. Orentreich and Durr. Mammogenesis in transsexuals.

26. Treves and Holleb. Cancer of the male breast.

27. Hoover, R., L. A. Gray, and B. MacMahon. 1976. Menopausal estrogens and breast cancer. *New Eng. J. Med.* 295:401.

28. Casagrande, J., U. Gerkins, et al. 1976. Exogenous estrogens and breast cancer in women with natural menopause. *J. Natl. Cancer Inst.* 56:839.

29. Burch, J., et al. 1975. The effects of long term estrogen therapy, estrogen in the postmenopause. *Front. Horm. Res.* 3:208.

30. Pike, M. C., et al. 1981. Oral contraceptive use and early abortion as risk factors for breast cancer in young women. *Br. J. Cancer* 43:72.

31. Paffenberger, R. S., et al. Cancer risk as related to use of oral contraceptives during fertile years. *Cancer* 39:1887.

32. Lees, A. W., et al. 1978. Oral contraceptives and breast disease in premenopausal Northern Alberta women. *Int. J. Cancer* 22:700.

33. Brinton, L. A., et al. 1979. Breast cancer risk factors among screening program participants. *J. Natl. Cancer Inst.* 62:37.

34. Pike et al. Oral contraceptive use.

35. Food and Drug Administration. Jan. 31, 1978. Drugs for human use: New drug requirements for labeling directed to the patient. Federal Register 43:4212.

12. GASTROINTESTINAL AND OTHER CANCERS

1. Rosen, P., S. M. Hellerstein, et al. 1981. The low incidence of colorectal cancer in a "high-risk" population. *Cancer* 48:2692.

2. Phillips, R. L. 1975. Role of life-style and dietary habits among Seventh-Day Adventists. *Cancer Res.* 35:3513.

3. Lyon, J. L., J. W. Gardner, et al. 1977. Low cancer incidence and mortality in Utah. *Cancer* 39:2608.

4. Wynder, E. L., et al. 1969. Environmental factors of cancer of the colon and rectum. II. Japanese epidemiological data. *Cancer* 32:1210.

5. Armstrong, B., and R. Doll. 1975. Environmental factors and cancer incidence and mortalities in different countries with special reference to dietary practices. *Int. J. Cancer* 15:617.

6. Burkitt, D. P. 1975. Large-bowel cancer: an epidemiological jigsaw puzzle. *J. Natl. Cancer Inst.* 54:3.

7. Haenszel, W. M., et al. 1973. Large bowel cancer in Hawaiian Japanese. *J. Natl. Cancer Inst.* 51:1765.

8. Aries, V. C., et al. 1969. Bacteria and the etiology of cancer of the large bowel. *Gut.* 10:334.

9. Miller, J. A., and E. C. Miller. 1969. The metabolic activation of carcinogenic aromatic amines and amides. *Prog. Exp. Tumor Res.* 11:273.

10. Maier, B., M. A. Flynn, et al. 1974. Effects of a high-beef diet on bowel-flora: a preliminary report. *Am. J. Clin. Nutr.* 27:1470.

11. Reddy, B. S., and T. Ohmori. 1981. Effect of intestinal microflora and dietary fat of 3,2^{1}-dimethyl-4-aminobiphenyl-induced colon carcinogenesis in F344 rats. *Cancer Res.* 41:1363.

12. Wynder, E. L., and B. S. Reddy. 1974. The epidemiology of cancer of the large bowel. *Digestive Diseases* 19:937.

13. Berg, J. W., M. A. Howell, and S. J. Silverman. 1973. Dietary hypothesis and diet related research in the etiology of colon cancer. *Health Serv. Reports* 88:915.

14. Hill, M. J., Drassar, et al. 1975. Fecal bile acids and clostridia in patients with cancer of the large bowel. *Lancet* 2:806.

15. Aries, V. C., et al. 1971. The effect of a strict vegetarian diet on the fecal flora and fecal steroid concentration. *J. Pathol.* 103:54.

16. MacDonald, I. A., et al. 1978. Fecal hydroxysteroid dehydrogenase activities in vegetarian Seventh-Day Adventists, control subjects, and bowel cancer patients. *Am. J. Clin. Nutr.* 31:S233.

17. Burkitt, D. P. 1971. Epidemiology of cancer of the colon and rectum. *Cancer* 28:3.

18. Hill, M. J., J. S. Crowther, et al. 1975. Bacteria and oetiology of cancer of the large bowel. *Lancet* 1:95.

19. Reddy, B. S., A. R. Hedges, et al. 1978. Metabolic epidemiology of large bowel cancer. Fecal bulk and constituents of high risk North American and low risk Finnish population. *Cancer* 42:2832.

20. *American Journal of Clinical Nutrition* 31 (suppl):512–20. Oct. 1978.

21. Eastwood, M. A. 1978. Fiber in the gastrointestinal tract. *Am. J. Clin. Nutr.* 31:30.

22. *Am. J. Clin. Nutr.* 31.

23. Ershoff, B. H. 1974. Antitoxic effects of plant fiber. *Am. J. Clin. Nutr.* 27:1395.

24. Phillips. Role of life-style and dietary habits.

25. Lyon, Gardner, et al. Low cancer incidence.

26. Burkitt. Large-bowel cancer.

27. Wynder and Reddy. Epidemiology of cancer.

28. Berg, Howell, and Silverman. Dietary hypothesis.

29. Hill, Drassar, et al. Fecal bile acids.

30. MacLennan, M. B., et al. 1978. Diet, transit time, stool weight, and colon cancer in two Scandinavian populations. *Am. J. Clin. Nutr.* 31:S239.

31. Graham, S., and C. Mettlin. 1979. Diet and colon cancer. *Am. J. Epidemiol.* 109:1.

32. Kritchevsky, D., and J. Story. 1974. Binding of bile salts *in vitro* by non-nutritive fiber. *J. Nutr.* 104:458.

33. Ibid.

34. Lai, C. 1978. Chlorophyll: the active factor in wheat sprout extract inhibiting the metabolic activation of carcinogens *in vitro. Nutr. Cancer* 1(3):19.

35. *Am. J. Clin. Nutr.* 31.

36. Burkitt, D. 1978. Colonic-rectal cancer: fiber and other dietary factors. *Am. J. Clin. Nutr.* 31:S58.

37. Jain, M., et al. 1980. A case control study of diet and colo-rectal cancer. *Int. J. Cancer* 26:757.

38. Gilbertsen, V. A., and J. M. Nelms. 1978. The prevention of invasive cancer of the rectum. *Cancer* 41:1137.

39. Gilbertsen, V. A. 1974. Protosigmoidoscopy and polypectomy in reducing the incidence of rectal cancer. *Cancer* 34:939.

40. Carroll, R. L., and M. Klein. 1980. How often should patients be sigmoidoscoped? *Prev. Med.* 9:741.

41. Larrson, L. A., A. Sandstrom, and P. Westling. 1975. Relationship of Plummer-Vinson disease to cancer of the upper alimentary tract in Sweden. *Cancer Res.* 35:3308.

42. Ibid.

43. Hirayama, T. 1979. Diet and cancer. *Nutrition and Cancer* 1(3):67.

44. Suzuki, K., and T. Mitsuoko. 1981. Increase in fecal nitrosamines in Japanese individuals given a Western diet. *Nature* 294:453.

45. Lee, D. H. K. 1970. Nitrates, nitrites, and methemoglobinemia. *Environ. Res.* 3:484.

46. Suzuki and Mitsuoko. Increase in fecal nitrosamines.

47. Hirayama. Diet and cancer.

48. Kriebel, D., and D. Jowett. 1980. Stomach mortality in the north central states: high risk is not limited to the foreign born. *Nutrition and Cancer* 1(2):8.

49. Armstrong and Doll. Environmental factors.

50. Ibid.

51. Polk, H. C. 1966. Carcinoma and the calcified gall bladder. *Gastroenterology* 50:582.

52. Bismuth, H., and R. A. Malt. 1979. Carcinoma of the biliary tract. *New Eng. J. Med.* 301:704.

53. Armstrong and Doll. Environmental factors.

54. MacMahon, B., S. Yen, et al. 1981. Coffee and cancer of the pancreas. *New Eng. J. Med.* 304:630.

55. Feinstein, A. R., et al. 1981. Coffee and pancreatic cancer. *JAMA* 246:957.

56. Goldstein, H. R. 1982. No association found between coffee and cancer of the pancreas. *New Eng. J. Med.* 306:997.

57. Armenian, H. K., et al. 1975. Epidemiologic characteristics of patients with prostatic neoplasms. *Am. J. Epidemiol.* 102:47.

58. Dunn, L. J., and J. T. Bradbury. 1967. Endocrine factors in endometrial carcinoma. *Am. J. Obstet. Gynecol.* 97:465.

59. Armstrong and Doll. Environmental factors.

60. Dunning, W. F., M. R. Curtis, and M. E. Maun. 1950. The effect of added dietary tryptophan on the occurrance of 2-acetylaminofluorene–induced liver and bladder cancers in rats. *Cancer Res.* 10:454.

61. Morrison, A. S., and J. E. Buring. 1980. Artificial sweeteners and cancer of the lower urinary tract. *New Eng. J. Med.* 302:537.

62. Hoover, R. N., and P. H. Strasser. 1980. Artificial sweeteners and human bladder cancer. *Lancet* (April):837.

63. Miller, A. B. 1977. The etiology of bladder cancer from the epidemiologic viewpoint. *Cancer Res.* 37:2929.

64. Hirayama. Diet and cancer.

65. Armstrong and Doll. Environmental factors.

66. Friedell, G. H., et al. 1979. Nutritional factors that may be involved in cancer of the bladder. *Nutrition and Cancer* 1(2):82.

67. Price, J. M. 1971. Etiology of bladder cancer. *In:* Benign and malignant tumors of the urinary bladder. E. Maltry, Jr. ed. Flushing, N.Y.: Med. Examination Publishing Co., Inc., 189–261.

68. Byar, D., and C. Blackard. 1977. Comparison of placebo, pyridoxine, and topical thiotepa in preventing recurrence of stage I bladder cancer. *Urology* 10:556.

69. Armstrong and Doll. Environmental factors.

70. Bjarnason, O., N. Day, et al. 1974. The effect of year of birth on the breast cancer age incidence curve in Iceland. *Int. J. Cancer* 13:689.

71. Workshop on fat and cancer. Sept. 1981. Supplement to *Cancer Res.* 41(9):3677.

72. Weisburger, J. H. 1979. Mechanism of action of diet as a carcinogen. *Cancer* 43:1987.

13. CARDIOVASCULAR DISEASE

1. Keys, A. 1970. Coronary heart disease in seven countries. *Circulation* 41(S):211.

2. Shekelle, R. B., et al. 1979. Diet, serum cholesterol, and death from coronary heart disease. *New Eng. J. Med.* 304:65.

3. Hjerman, I., et al. 1981. Effect of diet and smoking intervention on the incidence of coronary heart disease: Report from the Oslo study group of a randomized trial in healthy men. *Lancet* 2:1303.

4. Sacks, F. M., et al. 1981. Effect of ingestion of meat on plasma cholesterol of vegetarians. *JAMA* 246:640.

5. Gordon, T. 1970. The Framingham Diet Study: diet and regulation of serum cholesterol. *In:* Kannel, W. B., T. Gordon, eds. The Framingham Study: An epidemiological investigation of cardiovascular disease (Section 24). Washington, D.C.: Government Printing Office.

6. Pearce, M. L., and S. Dayton. 1971. Incidence of cancer in men on a diet high in polyunsaturated fat. *Lancet* i:464.

7. Ederer, F., P. Laren, et al. 1971. Cancer among men on cholesterol lowering diets. *Lancet* ii:203.

8. Rose, G., H. Blackburn, et al. 1974. Colon cancer and blood cholesterol. *Lancet* i:181.

9. Cambien, F., P. Ducimetetiere, and J. Richard. 1980. Total serum cholesterol and cancer mortality in a middle aged male population. *Am. J. Epidemiol.* 112:388.

10. Jain, M., et al. 1978. A case-control study of diet and colo-rectal cancer. *Int. J. Cancer* 26:757.

11. Dyerberg, J., H. O. Bang, et al. 1978. Eicosapenteanoic acid and prevention of thrombosis and atherosclerosis? *Lancet* 2:117; and *Lancet* 1980, 1:199.

12. Dyerberg, J., and H. O. Bang. 1979. Hemostatic function and platelet polyunsaturated fatty acids in Eskimos. *Lancet* 2:433.

13. Kobayashi, S., A. Hirai, et al. 1981. Reduction in blood viscosity by eicosapentaenoic acid. *Lancet* 2:197.

14. Conner, W. E., et al. 1981. The effects of eicosapentaenoic acid on blood lipids. *JAMA* 246:29.

15. Walker, A. R., and U. B. Arvidsson. 1954. Fat intake, serum cholesterol concentration and atherosclerosis in the South African Bantus. *J. Clin. Invest.* 33:1366.

16. Jenkins, D. J., et al. 1980. Dietary fiber and blood lipids: Treatment of hypercholesterolemia with guar crispbread. *Am. J. Clin. Nutr.* 33:575.

17. Ibid.

18. Gordon, T. The Framingham Diet Study.

19. Keys, A., C. Arvanis, et al. 1972. Coronary heart disease: overweight and obesity as risk factors. *Ann. Int. Med.* 77:15.

20. Dyer, A. R., J. Stamler, et al. 1975. Relationship of relative weight and body mass index to 14 year mortality in the Chicago People's Gas Co. study. *J. Chron. Dis.* 28:109.

21. Leon, A. S., and H. Blackburn. 1977. The relationship of physical activity to coronary heart disease and life expectancy. *Ann. N.Y. Acàd. Sci.* 301:561.

22. Stadel, B. V. 1981. Oral contraceptives and cardiovascular disease. *New Eng. J. Med.* 305:612.

23. Slone, D., et al. 1981. Risk of myocardial infarction in relation to current and discontinued use of oral contraceptives. *New Eng. J. Med.* 305:420.

24. Castelli, W. P., J. T. Doyle, et al. 1977. Alcohol and blood lipids. The Cooperative Lipoprotein Phenotyping Study. *Lancet* 2:153.

25. Yano, K., et al. 1977. Coffee, alcohol, and risk of coronary heart disease among Japanese men living in Hawaii. *New Eng. J. Med.* 297:405.

26. Henze, K., et al. 1977. Alcohol intake and coronary risk factors in a population group in Rome. *Nutr. Metab.* 21 Suppl 1:157.

27. Hulley, S. B., et al. 1977. Plasma high-density lipoprotein cholesterol level: influence of risk factor intervention. *JAMA* 238:2269.

28. Willett, W., et al. 1980. Alcohol consumption and high-density lipoprotein cholesterol in marathon runners. *New Eng. J. Med.* 303:1159.

14. EXERCISE AND RELAXATION

1. Hartung, H. G., J. Foreyt, et al. 1980. Relation of diet to high-density lipoprotein cholesterol in middle-aged marathon runners, joggers, and inactive men. *New Eng. J. Med.* 302:357.

2. Sylvester, R., J. Camp, and M. Sanonarco. 1977. Effects of exercise training on progression of documented coronary arteriosclerosis in men. *Ann. N.Y. Acad. Sci.* 301:495.

3. Gershbein, L. L., I. Benuck, and P. S. Shurrager. 1974. Influence of stress on lesion growth and on survival of animals bearing parenteral and intracerebral leukemia L1210 and Walker tumors. *Oncology* 30:429.

4. De Rosa, G., and N. R. Suarez. 1980. Effect of exercise on tumor growth and body composition of the host. *Fed. Am. Soc. Exp. Biol.* 1118.

5. Zeiner-Henrikson, T. 1976. Six year mortality related to cardiorespiratory symptoms and environmental risk factors in a sample of the Norwegian population. *J. Chron. Dis.* 29:15.

6. Paffenbarger, R. S., et al. 1978. Energy expenditure, cigarette smoking and blood pressure level as related to death from specific diseases. *Am. J. Epidemiol.* 108:12.

7. Pollack, M. L. 1973. The quantification and endurance training programs. *In:* Exercise and sport sciences reviews. Vol I. Wilmore, J. H., ed. New York: Academic Press.

8. Louis Harris and Associates, Inc. 1978. Perrier survey of fitness in America. Study No. S 2813. New York, N.Y.

9. Heald, F. 1975. Adolescent nutrition. *Med. Clin. North Am.* 59:1329.

10. Visintainer, M. A., et al. 1982. Tumor rejection in rats after inescapable or escapable shock. *Science* 216:437.

15. TEN-POINT PLAN FOR RISK FACTOR MODIFICATION

1. Korcok, M. 1981. Editorial. Pritikin vs. AHA diet: no difference for peripheral vascular disease. *JAMA* 246:1871.

2. Woolner, L. B., et al. 1981. Mayo Lung Project. Evaluation of lung cancer screening through Dec. 1979. *Mayo Clinic Proc.* 56:544.

Index

About the Author

Charles B. Simone, M.D., graduated from Rutgers Medical College and trained in internal medicine at the Cleveland Clinic. He then went to the National Cancer Institute of the National Institutes of Health in Bethesda, Maryland, and acquired training in medical oncology and clinical immunology. He is currently in the radiation therapy department at the Hospital of the University of Pennsylvania. During the past five years at the National Cancer Institute, Dr. Simone discovered the fundamental mechanism of how human white blood cells kill foreign cells. He also furthered the understanding of how complement proteins aid in killing. In addition, he developed a new treatment modality for killing cancer as well as infectious agents (called directed effector cells). He has tested this treatment in animals at the National Cancer Institute and will soon test it in cancer victims.